CELL BIOLOGY RESEARCH PROGRESS

DENDRITIC CELL BIOLOGY AS AN IMMUNE DYSFUNCTION IN NEOPLASIA

CELL BIOLOGY RESEARCH PROGRESS

Additional books and e-books in this series can be found on Nova's website under the Series tab.

CELL BIOLOGY RESEARCH PROGRESS

DENDRITIC CELL BIOLOGY AS AN IMMUNE DYSFUNCTION IN NEOPLASIA

LAWRENCE M. AGIUS

nova
Medicine & Health
New York

DOI: https://doi.org/10.52305/TJWV2594

Library of Congress Cataloging-in-Publication Data

ISBN: 978-1-68507-486-9

Published by Nova Science Publishers, Inc. † New York

Contents

PREFACE

This book deals with the susceptibility issues in the development of an effective response to antigenicity as presented by emerging or established neoplastic lesions. An attempt has been made to present critical views of the dysfunction of carcinogenesis in terms of evolving immune responses in terms of recruitment of dendritic cell biology. It is within such conceptual framework that autoimmunity presents an attractive response to neoplasia in terms that allow for access to the malignant transformation process. It is significant to potentiate the immune responses that involve the integral immune dimensions that characterize and recharacterize the dynamics of turnover of dendritic cells as the most powerful agents in presentation of neoantigenicity as provided by tumor cell proliferation and spread within the body.

The performance of staged dimensions in antigen exposure by tumor cells is critical to the presentation of tumor cells as brought forward by the proposed dynamics of an interface between tumor cells and the tumor microenvironment in the realization of an extensive autoimmune response with the realization of performance exposure of the antigenicity as a biologic agent in its own right.

This book is aimed to cancer researchers and pathologists and immunologists with a strong interest in carcinogenesis and cancer cell progression as dictated by proposed immune response to tumor antigenicity.

Chapter 1

Active Participation of Dendritic Cells in Tumor Cell Immune Evasion

Abstract

Conveying influences of a dual participation of dendritic cells and of tumor cells emerge in the shaping and reshaping of phenotype characterization of the high degree of plasticity attributes of dendritic cells (DC) in particular. In such terms, DC come to play an active essential role of the tumor cell evasion of the immune response that is transferable in terms of the contextual influences and modulations, as defined by immature versus mature stage specificities of the dendritic cells. In terms that go beyond such considerations, the incremental responses of intracellular mediators within both dendritic cells and tumor cells convey a realization that involves, in inherent manner, the evasion of the tumor cells from the immunosurveillance programs otherwise projected by dendritic cells.

Introduction

Signaling pathways in both tumor cells and dendritic cells (DC) constitute a predominant system series of inhibitors in suppressing immunosurveillance of tumors. In such manner, inhibitors of p38 MAPK,

JAK/STAT3, PI3K/Akt and NF kappaB constitute possible mechanisms as target molecular pathways in enhancing differentiation and functional activity in DC.

Transforming growth factor (TGF)-beta is central to immune suppression with roles in tutor immune evasion and poor responses to cancer immunotherapy [1].

The constitutive mechanistic pathways of tumor cells involve the secretion of various cytokines such as IL-6, IL-10, and TGF- beta, as after the exposure of DC to tumor culture-conditioned medium and inhibitors or antibodies against these specific cytokines that restore differentiation and functionality of DC against tumor cells. Natural Killer cells stimulate DC recruitment into the tumor microenvironment, enhancing cancer immune control; a cellular and molecular checkpoint for intratumoral DC recruitment is targeted by tumor-derived prostaglandin E2 for immune evasion [2].

INTRACELLULAR PATHWAYS

Such considerations incorporate the essential roles of intracellular pathway mechanisms in the tumor cell evasion of immune response pathway dynamics of DC. Mechanisms are utilised by cancers to induce DC toleration, with various parallels between the evolution of these mechanisms and the process of mesenchymal transformation involved in tumorigenesis and metastasis [3]. In such terms, ongoing derivative dimensions of intracellular signaling may be transferable factors in the evolutionary history of tumor cell evasion from the immunosurveillance programs as conveyed by DC. The causes of breast cancer's immune silence derive from mechanisms that diminish immune recognition and others that promote strong immunosuppression [4].

An essential feature of tumor evasion is the effect of secreted soluble factors that tumor cells produce in the abrogation of the immune response as resulting from impaired differentiation and maturation of DC from bone marrow hematopoietic progenitor cells and monocytes. In such terms, ongoing system profile derivation is intrinsic historic role for the activation of antitumor immune responses.

The depiction of area and regional systems is conveyed especially by the localization of DC in peripheral tissues that reach regional lymph nodes in the differentiation programs undergone by circulating DC. It is significant to view DC participatory roles in immunosurveillance as target inhibition by evading tumor cells. New immune therapies are able to reverse immune evasion strategies of tumor cells, with also the blockade of immune checkpoints cytotoxic T-lymphocyte antigen 4 and programmed death-1 [5].

STAGE DEPENDENCE

Stage dependence of p38 MAPK (Mitogen activated protein kinase) is illustrated by inhibition of DC differentiation and maturation when DC is derived from monocytes. The incremental dimensions of such stage-dependence is assumed within the context of the need for p38 MAPK in the generation of immature DC to form mature and cytokine-secreting DC. It is significant to recognize the plasticity of DC as conveyed by stage-dependence in the maturation of immunosurveillance programs, in response to a multitude of evading systems as transferable Microsystems carried forward by tumor cells. The programmed cell death protein 1 pathway plays a role in eliciting the immune checkpoint response of T cells and application of anti-PD-1/PD-L1 antibodies as checkpoint inhibitors are rapidly becoming a promising therapeutic approach [6].

It is further to such conditioned mediators produced by tumor cells that DC play also active roles in tumor evasion by means of manipulated maturational context as transferred by immature DC. In such terms, ongoing programs of interaction of immature DC and of actively proliferating cells include various intracellular signaling pathways that are stage-dependent. Mechanisms have evolved in cancers to alter DC metabolic pathways, thus allowing for continued tumor progression and metastasis [7].

Myeloma Patients

In myeloma patients, mature DC produce significantly less CD1a, CD40, CD80 and HLA-DR and are poor in activating autologous antigen-specific T cells. Such phenomena are indicative of a transforming series of activities that are derived from interactivities of DC with tumor cells. The attributes of such interactivities between DC and tumor cells may be conveyed by elevated production of such autologous cytokines as represented by IL-6, activated p38 MAPK and STAT3, and inhibited MEK/ERK signaling pathways in DC progenitor cells.

The immunosuppressive tumor microenvironment is a major barrier to immunotherapy and tumor-derived retinoid acid regulates intratumor monocyte differentiation to enhance immune suppression [8].

Reprogramming

Attenuation of regulatory T cells in response to Toll-like receptor agonists results from inhibiting p38 MAPK signaling. Thus, inhibiting p38 MAPK by SB203580 allows for the emergence of promoted type 1 T cell responses. An understanding of the differential maturation steps of DC may help clarify the mechanisms of initial commitment of tumor cells that are involved in the emergence of either Th1 or Th2 subsets. ERK inhibition is also a potential target mechanism for contextual evasion of the tumor cells from the immune system response.

Dendritic Cell Maturation

JAK/STAT3 signaling pathways are also inhibiting systems in DC maturation, and as such, are instrumental in further conditioning the antitumor immune response.

Cross-talk with the NF kappaB on the part of JAK/STAT, p38 MAPK and ERK signaling pathways potentiates the transcription programs of target genes, such as the expression of IL-12. A significant correlate is the high level of activity of NF kappaB in tumor-induced DC dysfunction in patients with cancer.

One essential mechanism behind CD47-mediated immune evasion is interaction with signals regulatory protein-alpha (SIRPalpha) expressed on myeloid cells; this induces phosphorylation of SIRPalpha cytoplasmic immunoreceptor tyrosine-based inhibition motifs and recruitment of Src homology 2 domain-containing tyrosine phosphatases to ultimately result in delivering an anti-phagocytic-signal [9].

Specifically High Levels of Signaling

High levels of signaling pathway mediators are a specific mechanism in the deregulating of maturation programs that result specifically in tumor evasion of the immune system responses. As such, hyperactivation of key signaling pathways is parent mechanism in the deregulation of the interacting dynamics of the DC with tumor cells, as these latter produce and maintain contextual evasion from the immune response.

Preclinical data show that inhibition of cyclooxygenase synergizes with anti-PD-1 blockade in inducing tumor eradication, thus suggesting that COX inhibitors may be useful adjuvants in immunotherapy of tumor patients [10]. Recent preclinical data suggest new therapies to subvert tutor induced immunosuppression via prostaglandin inhibition [11].

Conclusion

A scenario of interactivities of DC with tumor cells emerges as terms of reference of intracellular signaling pathways in both DC and malignant cells.

In such context, the differential status of maturation stages of DC and the high levels of these mediators are central contextual conditioning systems acquired by tumor cells that target and abrogate the antitumor immune response.

In a final analysis maturation of DC is a functional correlate of the intracellular signaling pathways within both DC and tumor cells, as these two cell types interact to derail the system profiles of the central roles of the immunosurveillance mechanisms. Abnormal DC differentiation, hence, is a corollary phenomenon in DC active participation, inducing immune response evasion, as also instigated by the tumor cells. The contextual references of such a concept is inherent derivative for the active participation of DC in provoking a sustained tumor evasion in terms of the high degree of plasticity, as evidenced by the sharp dichotomy between roles played, respectively, by immature versus mature DC phenotypes.

References

[1] Batlle E, Massague J "Transforming Growth Factor-beta signaling in immunity and cancer" *Immunity* 2019;50(4):924-940.

[2] Bottcher JP, Bonavita E, Chakravarty P, Blees H, Cabeza-Cabrerizo M, Sammicheli S et al. "NK cells stimulate recruitment of cDC1 into the tumor microenvironment promoting cancer immune control" *Cell* 2018;172(5):1022-1037.

[3] DeVito NC, Plebanek MP, Theivanthiran B, Hanks BA "Role of tumor-mediated dendritic cell tolerization in in immune evasion" *Front Immune* 2019;10:2876.

[4] Bates JP, Derakhshandeh R, Jones L, Webb TJ "Mechanisms of immune evasion in breast cancer" *BMC Cancer* 2018;18(1):556.

[5] Muenst S, Laubli H, Soysal SD, Zippelius A, Tzankov A, Hoeller S "The immune system and cancer evasion strategies: therapeutic concepts" *J Intern Med* 2016;279(6):541-62.

[6] Wu X, Gu Z, Chen Y, Chen B, Chen W, Weng L et al. "Application of PD-1 blockade in cancer immunotherapy" *Comput Struct Biotechnol J* 2019/17:661-674.
[7] Plebanek MP, Sturdivant M, DeVito NC, Hanks BA "Role of dendritic cell metabolic reprogramming in tumor immune evasion" *Int Immune* 2020;32(7):485-491.
[8] Devalaraja S, To TKJ, Folkert IW, Natesan R, Alam MZ, Li M et al. "Tumor-derived retinoic acid regulates intratumor monocyte differentiation to promote immune suppression" *Cell* 2020;180(6):1098-1114.
[9] Liu X, Kwon H, Li Z, Fu YX "Is CD47 an innate immune checkpoint for tumor evasion?" *J Hematol Oncol* 2017;10(1):12.
[10] Zelenay S, van der Veen AG, Bottcher JP, Snelgrove KJ, Rogers N, Acton SE et al. "Cycloosygenase-dependent tumor growth through evasion of immunity" *Cell* 2015;162(6):1257-70.
[11] Wang D, DuBois RN "The role of prostaglandin E(2) in tumor-associated immunosuppression" *Trends Mol Med* 2016;22(1):1-3.

Chapter 2

AGING-INDUCED ABERRANT DENDRITIC CELLS IN TERMS OF HIGHLY PROLIFERATIVE TUMOR CELL CLONAL SUBSETS

ABSTRACT

The system profiles of incongruent equilibrating phenomena of direct cell to cell contact are inherent attributes of interactivity as redefined with respect to innate and adaptive co-operability. In such terms, ongoing proliferation of tumor cell subsets is provocative dimension of a parent phenomenon of induction of the immune response. Immunosurveillance pathways of cell contact and adhesion are participant partners within a system of aging of the DC, as borne out by the operative exposure of tumor neoantigens. It is significant to view the parent inducing phenomenon as one that arises within the highly proliferative clones of tumor cells projected, in turn, by the distributional biology of a pressure immunity. The creation of neoantigenicity is itself an actively inducing dimension for further proliferation and spread of the proliferating tumor clones of spread.

INTRODUCTION

The effects of aging on dendritic cell numbers and function operate at multiple levels of induction of T lymphocytes. Mechanical tension in a tissue microenvironment is a critical environmental cue of DC (dendritic cells) and innate immunity; tension identifies the Hippo-signaling molecule TAZ as well as Ca2+related ion channels including potentially PIEZO1, and primes DC to elicit an adaptive immune response [1]. The important constituents comprising regulatory T cells is one facet in the overall immunity related to naïve T cell activation. In such terms, multiple defects in DC responsiveness, in the employment of DC vaccination, are reported as linked to bone marrow progenitor recruitment in particular. The distributional biology of migration of DC cells is inherently linked to maturation of these professional antigen-presenting cells. Impaired dendritic cell function in raging promotes defective antitumor immunity [2]. The further conformational dimensions of aging relate to the prominent roles of the DC in a manner that potentially impacts targeting of naïve T lymphocytes.

DISTRIBUTIONAL BIOLOGY

Distributional biology of DC is associated with the targeting of T cells as dictated largely by specific chemokine actions. In terms of derivatively operative activation of the T-cell immune response lies within the system operability of a generic induction phenomenon.

In relative relationship to such processes, it is significant to consider aging as a constitutively performing operability that relates to the exposure of often old DC subset response at multiple levels of DC dysfunction. The further incremental response of young DC is highly dependent on the emergence of co-stimulatory molecules on the surface of these cells. Immune gene signature defines a subclass of thyroid cancer with poor clinical outcomes [3]. Significant cooperative dimensions are potentially target organ responsiveness in a manner that determines the immune responsiveness of the elderly patient population.

Lymphatic endothelial cells regulate immune responses by affecting entry of immune cells into lymphatic capillaries, presenting antigens on major histocompatibility complex proteins and modulating antigen presenting cells; subtle forms of lymphatic injury may occur in raging and in the tumor microenvironment [4].

INFLAMMATORY CYTOKINES

Paradoxical dimensions of the inflammatory cytokines of the TNF factor superfamily and other factors including lipopolysaccharides induce and further redefine such induction of a T-lymphocyte response. Such response incorporates both cytotoxic and helper T cell subpopulations in a manner of a series of interactions as dominantly determined, in particular, by regulatory T lymphocytes.

Innate and adaptive immune responses constitute different subpopulations of incremental potential towards the attainment of DC vaccination effectiveness.

The distributional biology of DC is inherently a product of the continuous process of their maturation, as also within the responsiveness of old DC subsets. Although DC immunotherapy primarily targets the elderly, little is known about the impact of aging on DC functions [5].

INDUCTION

Paradoxymal dimensions of operative induction thus signify the emergence of systems of response within further dimensions of interaction of old DC with various levels of significant participation as dictated by the aging process. Wnt signaling is implicated in age-associated diseases such as cancer and is important in maintaining tissue homeostasis [6]. The involvement of aging as determinant in potential induction of the antitumor immune response participates with the parent malignant transformation phenomenon. In such terms, multiple levels of exposure to pathogen associated molecular patterns are inducing phenomena in a manner that redefines biology of DC defects in an antitumor response.

As the most potent antigen presenting cells, DC are capable of sensitising T cells to new and recall antigens [7]. The incremental overall participation in defining the nature of the immune responsiveness to tumor antigenicity is intrinsic component acquisition of maturation of the DC, as often seen in various tumor bearing animals.

Inflammatory responsiveness is intrinsic component participation of the antitumor immune reactivity within equilibrating dimensions for further compromise of the tumor cells and of their inherent antigenicity as presented to DC and T cell populations. In such terms, induction of the immune response is itself a multi-layer phenomenon within the contextual setting for tumor population elimination. Recent studies suggest that the antitumor immune response is reduced in both aging and obesity, while responsiveness to immune checkpoint blockade is paradoxically intact [8]. Such redefining parameters operate as system profiles that induce especially regulatory T cells.

The hallmarks of immunosenescence include reduced numbers of naive CD4+ and CD8+ T cells, an imbalance in T cell subsets and diminished T cell receptor repertoire and signaling; myeloid-derived suppressor cells appear potent inducers of immunosenescence [9]. The participation of aberrant DC responses with aging is significant in terms of the ongoing induction process of antigen presentation to both the innate and adaptive immune responses. The aging process is itself redefined within the proliferation and maturation phenomena of DC. The further conformational roles of the aberrant DC are contextual reference to a sustained effort to induced response. Immunosenescence appears to be caused by an increased activity of immunosuppressive cells rather than cellular senescence [10].

Performance Dynamics

Performance dynamics of DC aging is a contextual restriction of the antitumor response in a manner that participates as defined induction of T-lymphocyte reactivation.

Immature myeloid-derived suppressor cells play a crucial role in the immune escape of tumor cells [11]. The terms of such aberrant operability are therefore a response of the immune system as categorized within the antigen-exposure phenomenon itself. DC are substantial evidence for antigen exposure that is defined by the nature of tumor cell proliferation and spread. The DC migrate within terms of reference of systems of metastasis potentiality. The incremental elements of an antitumor immune response are resultant operability of the inherent nature of aging DC, and of a constitutive process of interaction of various DC subsets as strictly equilibrating processes of induction and of response. The co-operation between senescent cells and immunosuppressive MDSCs regulates not only carcinogenesis and chronic inflammatory disorders but may promote the low-grade chronic inflammation in the aging process [12]. Immunosenescence includes remodelling of lymphoid organs with altered immune function in the early and is closely related to infections, autoimmune diseases and cancer [13].

Induction of functional tumor-specific CD8+ cytotoxic T lymphocytes is the ultimate aim of all immunotherapies [14].

Conclusion

Dimensions of operability in terms of an antitumor immune response is intrinsic attribute for the involvement of antigen exposure, as itself defined by the nature of the carcinogenesis process of tumor proliferation and spread.

The involvement of aging as prescribed within systems of potential induction of the immune response to tumors is inherent redefining terms of the status of immune response of the aging patient. In such terms, ongoing processes of maturation of DC are related intrinsically to the aging cancer patient as well projected by inducing phenomena of antigen exposure by proliferating and spreading tumor cells. It is significant to view substantial responses to tumor neoantigenicity as defined restriction processes of redefined tumor cell processes of induced cell-to-cell contact, as orchestrated by DC. Performance dynamics are hence pressure immunity phenomena that signify the immune surveillance of the aging patient population.

In such terms, the further participation of the immune system is equilibrating interactivity of the innate with the adaptive immune systems. The operability of response to tumor neoantigenicity is also dysfunction of antigen exposure by highly proliferative tumor cell subsets.

REFERENCES

[1] Chakraborty M, Chu K, Shrestha A, Revelo XS, Zhang X, Gold MJ et al. "Mechanical stiffness controls dendritic cell metabolism and function" *Cell Rep* 2021;34(2):108609.

[2] Grolleau-Julius A, Harning EK, Abernathy LM, Yung RL "Impaired dendritic cell function in aging leads to defective antitumor immunity" *Cancer Res* 2008;68(15):6341-9.

[3] Zhi J, Yi J, Tian M, Wang H, Kang N, Zheng X et al. "Immune gene signature delineates a subclass of thyroid cancer with unfavourable clinical outcomes" *Aging* (Albany NY) 2020;12(7):5733-5750.

[4] Kataru RP, Baik JE, Park HJ, Wiser I, Rehal S, Shin JY et al. "Regulation of immune function by the lymphatic system in lymphedema" *Front Immune* 2019;10:470.

[5] Grolleau-Julius A, Garg MR, Mo R, Stoolman LL, Yung RL "Effect of aging on bone marrow-derived murine CD11c+CD4-CD8alpha dendritic cell function" *J Gerontol A Biol Sci Med Sci* 2006;61(10):1039-47.

[6] Garcia-Velazquez L, Arias C "The emerging role of Wnt signaling dysregulation in the understanding and modification of age-associated diseases" *Ageing Res Rev* 2017;37:135-145.

[7] Grolleau-Julius A, Abernathy L, Harning E, Yung RL "Mechanisms of murine dendritic cell antitumor dysfunction in aging" *Cancer Immune Immuother* 2009;58(12):1935-9.

[8] Drijvers JM, Sharpe AH, Haigis MC "The effects of waging and systemic metabolism on antitumor T cell responses" *Elife* 2020;9:e62420/

[9] Salminen A, Kaarniranta K, Kauppinen A "Immunosenescence: the potential role of myeloid-derived suppressor cells (MDSC) in age-related immune deficiency" *Cell Mol Life Sci* 2019;76(10):1901-1918.

[10] Salminen A "Activation of immunosuppressive network in the raging process" *Ageing Res Rev* 2020;57:100998.

[11] Salminen A, Kaarniranta K, Kauppinen A "Phytochemicals inhibit the immunosuppressive functions of myeloid-derived suppressor cells (MDSC): impact on cancer and age-related chronic inflammatory disorders" *Int Immunopharmacol* 2018;61:231-240.

[12] Salminen A, Kauppinen A, Kaarniranta K "Myeloid-derived suppressor cells (MDSC): an important partner in cellular/tissue senescence" *Biogerontology* 2018;19(5):325-339.

[13] Lian J, Yue Y, Yu W, Zhang Y "Immunosenescence: a key player in cancer development" *J Hematol Oncol* 2020;13(1):151.

[14] Huff WX, Kwon JH, Henriquez M, Fetcko K, Dey M "The evolving role of CD8+ CD28- immunosenescent T cells in cancer immunology" *Int J Sci* 2019:20(11):2810.

Chapter 3

SUSTAINED METABOLIC SYSTEM IMBALANCE AS INDUCED IMMUNE SUPPRESSION OF DENDRITIC CELLS IN TUMOR NEOANTIGENICITY PROFILES

ABSTRACT

The conformity events within defined pathways of immune suppression are significant as further proposed by the emergence of tolerogenicity and as further documented by tumor cell proliferation and progression. In such series of phenomena, the dendritic cells both induce and further incorporate the events of contact inhibition within realized metabolic intermediates of the kynunerine pathway. The embodiment of descriptive biologic events as compounded in projected induction is integral to the network nature of immune responsiveness and also to the induction of immune tolerance. In such terms, ongoing pathways of non-resolution are integral systems as metabolic intermediates accumulate principally within the dendritic cells as principal antigen-presenting cells. The conclusive formats, as proposed, are independent of the various intermediate pathways of such non-resolution of tumor neoantigenicity.

The proposed active effect of tumor antigenicity is integral to a further projected series of tryptophan starvation as proposed within integral networks for immune suppression.

INTRODUCTION

Indoleamine pyrrole 2,3 dioxygenase (IDO) is recognized as inducing tryptophan starvation and in generating metabolite toxic effects which act on T lymphocytes and also in generating regulatory T cells. Such phenomena are cardinal dimensional effectors within the further induced suppression of T lymphocyte cell arrest in the mid G1 phase and even as induced apoptosis of T cells. Tumor infiltrating lymphocytes therapy for ovarian appears at the point of translation, requiring combined methodologies [1].

The central assumed dysfunctions of such IDO action are imbalance events within the evolutionary dimensions of injury as induced by a minor population subset of dendritic cells (DC). These are expounded by the activities intrinsic to antigen presentation. In such terms, the ongoing participation of the suppressive effects of IDO and its metabolites includes the evolutionary emergence of injury to the T lymphocytes within a contextual framework of both T4+ and T8+ lymphocytes.

In such manner, the incremental dimensions of ongoing suppressive effects of the antitumor immune response incriminate a whole series of events within system biology of DC. It is further to such considerations that derivative contexts of an immune response to cancer cells induce the further inherent dimensions for further suppression of the antitumor response. The ability of Natural Killer cells to bridge innate and "downstream" adaptive immune responses renders them an ideal platform to base new cancer therapeutics [2].

INCREMENTAL PARAMETERS

Incremental parameters of a positive feedback response operating on actions of antigen presentation by DC incriminate the T lymphocytes and Natural Killer cells within encompassed revenues for cell division suppression as projected by the action of IDO+ DC. IDO induces T cell exhaustion and increased generation of regulatory T cells, up-regulating expression of inhibitory receptors and ligands [3]. Integral effects of immune suppression are propagating influence in terms of DC dimensions, as further projected within limits of tolerogenic influence as exerted by regulatory DC.

In terms of ongoing dynamics of DC mobility and trafficking to tumor draining lymph nodes, the further suppression on T lymphocytes is exemplified by the propagation of DC within system profile of such events depicted principally by eventual lymphocyte apoptosis. An effective response to anti-programmed cell death ligand 1/programmed cell death 1 therapy depends on establishing an integrated immune cycle, and combination with epigenetic agents my retrain the immune system [4].

NEOANTIGENICITY

Conclusive formulations of immune suppression allow a permissive tolerance to tumor neoantigenicity, as provided by the inclusive frameworks for further events as effected by DC. The whole integrating interactions of DC are further compounding systems of response, on the one hand, and of a tolerogenicity that derives from IDO+ DC action.

The foregoing dimensions incorporate a strong susceptibility to the ongoing foreplay of molecular components of both soluble and insoluble pathway metabolites of the kynurenine pathway.

In realization of such events, the incorporation of derivatives would include the development of suppression as projected by tolerogenicity by T lymphocytes of regulatory functionality. The incorporation of serial exposure to neoantigens is compound phenomenon within systems of biologic determinism, as further propounded by immune privilege and immune tolerance. In such terms, ongoing metabolic consequences of tryptophan starvation are cardinal events as proposed by pathway metabolite imbalance down-stream to tryptophan insufficiency. A chemo-immunotherapy approach utilises a liposomal carrier to simultaneously trigger immunogenic cell death as well as interfere in the regionally over expressed immunosuppression due to IDO at the breast cancer tumor site [5].

The generic compounding influence of IDO + DC is necessarily complex reformulation of the tumor antigenicities themselves. In such terms ongoing corporative dimensions include the derivative regulatory DC within systems for further suppressive influence. In animal tumor models, genetic or pharmacological IDO1 inhibition can induce the (re)activation of antitumor immune responses [6].

IDO is a central feature of DC action with regulatory function both in cancer and chronic infection; a link exists between tuuor necrosis factor alpha, prostaglandin E2 and IDO [7].

The proposed realization of cell injury to T lymphocytes is central to further co-operative events, as propounded by the incremental induction of a tolerance that bespeaks of dimensions of projection of immune suppression by systems of receptor and effector modalities. Analysis of plasma kynurenine/tryptophan levels in patients with cancer confirms that the IDO pathway is activated in several types of cancer [8]. The ongoing realizations of system pathways are further context for the emergence of significance in the ongoing participation of T lymphocyte injury. Besides targeting tumor antigens and inducing tumor cell death, tumor antigen-targeting monoclonal antibodies interact with immune cells through Fc-dependent mechanisms to induce adaptive memory immune responses [9].

IMMUNE TOLERANCE

The significance of immune tolerance is further projected by models of tumor progression within the system profiles of induction, and also non-induction, of pathways of metabolic co-operativity. In such terms, ongoing events incorporate the proposed pathway nomogram as induced by intermediates of such pathways. The induction of actual dimensions are contextual conformity within systems of response, and also nonresponse, to tumor neoantigenicity. The magnitude and the type of immune response depends on the local cytokine milieu and the aryl hydrocarbon receptor is one key factor involved in the fine-tuning of this cytokine balance [10].

In terms that bespeak of such inducive actions, the property realization of T lymphocyte response is cardinal consideration within systems as projected within frameworks for further development of immune tolerance to tumor neoantigenicity.

CONCLUSION

The conclusive phenomena that contribute to a sustained immunologic tolerance are derivative metabolite system series that incorporate the compound profiles for further generation of immune suppression. IDO is over expressed in both cancer cells and antigen-presenting cells in tumor-draining lymph nodes where it promotes peripheral immune tolerance to tumor antigens; inhibitors of IDO reverse this immunosuppression, complementing classical cytotoxic cancer chemotherapy [11]. In such terms, the contextual cellular contact events are also persistent inducing series of influences that partake as further phenomena of sustainment biology mechanics. The proposed incorporation of antigenicity as foreign elements is well exemplified by the infectious and parasitic dimensions of such antigen exposure. In the case of tumors, the co-operative performance of dimensionality is proposed sustainment of such antigen exposure as provided by pathway metabolic events. The proposed significance of such phenomena is inducing influence per se as proposed by tumor antigenicity.

Further idealization formulas are pathway-derived within the compounding effects of events primarily of antigenicity-suppressive action in generating tolerogenicity.

REFERENCES

[1] Santoiemma PP, Powell DJ Jr "Tumor infiltrating lymphocytes in ovarian cancer" *Cancer Biol There* 2015;16(6):807-20.

[2] Pockley AG, Vaupel P, Multhoff G "NK cell-based therapeutics for lung cancer" *Expert Opin Biol There* 2020;30(1):23-33.

[3] Liu M, Li Ziyang, Yao W, Zeng X, Wang L, Cheng J et al "IDO inhibitor synergised with radiotherapy to delay tumor growth by reversing T cell exhaustion" *Mol Med Rep* 2020;21(1):445-453.

[4] Chen X, Pan X, Zhang W, Guo H, Cheng S, He Q et al. "Epigenetic strategies synergies with PD-L1/PD-1 targeted cancer immunotherapies to enhance antitumor responses" *Acta Pharm Sin* B 2020;10(5):723-733.

[5] Lu J, Liu X, Liao YP, Wang X, Ahmed A, Jiang W et al. "Breast cancer chemo-immunotherapy through liposomal delivery of an immunogenic cell death stimulus plus interference in the IDO-1 pathway" *ACS Nano* 2018;12(11):11041-11061.

[6] Le Naour J, Galluzzi L, Zitvogel L, Kroemer G, Vacchelli E "Trial watch: IDO inhibitors in cancer therapy" *Oncoimmunology* 2020;9(1):1777625.

[7] Popov A, Schultze JL "IDO-expressing regulatory dendritic cells in cancer and chronic infection" *J Mol Med* (Berl) 2008;86(2):145-60.

[8] Liu X, Shin N, Koblish HK, Yang G, Wang Q, Wang K et al. "Selective inhibition of IDO1 effectively regulates mediators of antitumor immunity" *Blood* 2019;115(17):3520-30.

[9] Michaud HA, Eliaou JF, Lafont V, Bonnefoy N, Gros L "Tumor antigen-targeting monoclonal antibody-based immunotherapy: orchestrating combined strategies for the development of long-term antitumor immunity" *Oncoimmunology* 2014;3(9):e955684.

[10] Hao N, Whitelaw ML "The emerging roles of AhR in physiology and immunity" *Biochem Pharmacy* 2013;86(5):561-70.

[11] Katz JB, Muller AJ, Prendergast GC "Indoleamine 2,3-dioxygenase in T-cell tolerance and tumor immune escape" *Immune Rev* 2008;222:206-21.

Chapter 4

INCLUSIVE LOSS OF INTEGRITY OF THE ANTITUMOR IMMUNE RESPONSE AS CHEMOKINE PATTERNS OF NONRECOGNITION

ABSTRACT

The conformity events within defined pathways of immune suppression are significant as further proposed by the emergence of tolerogenicity and as further documented by tumor cell proliferation and progression. In such series of phenomena, the dendritic cells both induce and further incorporate the events of contact inhibition within realized metabolic intermediates of the kynunerine pathway. The embodiment of descriptive biologic events as compounded in projected induction is integral to the network nature of immune responsiveness and also to the induction of immune tolerance. In such terms, ongoing pathways of non-resolution are integral systems as metabolic intermediates accumulate principally within the dendritic cells as principal antigen-presenting cells. The conclusive formats, as proposed, are independent of the various intermediate pathways of such non-resolution of tumor neoantigenicity.

The proposed active effect of tumor antigenicity is integral to a further projected series of tryptophan starvation as proposed within integral networks for immune suppression.

Introduction

Indoleamine pyrrole 2,3 dioxygenase (IDO) is recognized as inducing tryptophan starvation and in generating metabolite toxic effects which act on T lymphocytes and also in generating regulatory T cells. Such phenomena are cardinal dimensional effectors within the further induced suppression of T lymphocyte cell arrest in the mid G1 phase and even as induced apoptosis of T cells. Tumor infiltrating lymphocytes therapy for ovarian appears at the point of translation, requiring combined methodologies [1].

The central assumed dysfunctions of such IDO action are imbalance events within the evolutionary dimensions of injury as induced by a minor population subset of dendritic cells (DC). These are expounded by the activities intrinsic to antigen presentation.

In such terms, the ongoing participation of the suppressive effects of IDO and its metabolites includes the evolutionary emergence of injury to the T lymphocytes within a contextual framework of both T4+ and T8+ lymphocytes. In such manner, the incremental dimensions of ongoing suppressive effects of the antitumor immune response incriminate a whole series of events within system biology of DC. It is further to such considerations that derivative contexts of an immune response to cancer cells induce the further inherent dimensions for further suppression of the antitumor response. The ability of Natural Killer cells to bridge innate and "downstream" adaptive immune responses renders them an ideal platform to base new cancer therapeutics [2].

Incremental Parameters

Incremental parameters of a positive feedback response operating on actions of antigen presentation by DC incriminate the T lymphocytes and Natural Killer cells within encompassed revenues for cell division suppression as projected by the action of IDO+ DC.

IDO induces T cell exhaustion and increased generation of regulatory T cells, up-regulating expression of inhibitory receptors and ligands [3]. Integral effects of immune suppression are propagating influence in terms of DC dimensions, as further projected within limits of tolerogenic influence as exerted by regulatory DC. In terms of ongoing dynamics of DC mobility and trafficking to tumor draining lymph nodes, the further suppression on T lymphocytes is exemplified by the propagation of DC within system profile of such events depicted principally by eventual lymphocyte apoptosis. An effective response to anti-programmed cell death ligand 1/programmed cell death 1 therapy depends on establishing an integrated immune cycle, and combination with epigenetic agents my retrain the immune system [4].

NEOANTIGENICITY

Conclusive formulations of immune suppression allow a permissive tolerance to tumor neoantigenicity, as provided by the inclusive frameworks for further events as effected by DC.

The whole integrating interactions of DC are further compounding systems of response, on the one hand, and of a tolerogenicity that derives from IDO+ DC action.

The foregoing dimensions incorporate a strong susceptibility to the ongoing foreplay of molecular components of both soluble and insoluble pathway metabolites of the kynurenine pathway. In realization of such events, the incorporation of derivatives would include the development of suppression as projected by tolerogenicity by T lymphocytes of regulatory functionality. The incorporation of serial exposure to neoantigens is compound phenomenon within systems of biologic determinism, as further propounded by immune privilege and immune tolerance. In such terms, ongoing metabolic consequences of tryptophan starvation are cardinal events as proposed by pathway metabolite imbalance down-stream to tryptophan insufficiency. A chemo-immunotherapy approach utilises a liposomal carrier to simultaneously trigger immunogenic cell death as well as interfere in the regionally over expressed immunosuppression due to IDO at the breast cancer tumor site [5].

The generic compounding influence of IDO + DC is necessarily complex reformulation of the tumor antigenicities themselves. In such terms ongoing corporative dimensions include the derivative regulatory DC within systems for further suppressive influence. In animal tumor models, genetic or pharmacological IDO1 inhibition can induce the (re)activation of antitumor immune responses [6]. IDO is a central feature of DC action with regulatory function both in cancer and chronic infection; a link exists between tuuor necrosis factor alpha, prostaglandin E2 and IDO [7].

The proposed realization of cell injury to T lymphocytes is central to further co-operative events, as propounded by the incremental induction of a tolerance that bespeaks of dimensions of projection of immune suppression by systems of receptor and effector modalities. Analysis of plasma kynurenine/tryptophan levels in patients with cancer confirms that the IDO pathway is activated in several types of cancer [8]. The ongoing realizations of system pathways are further context for the emergence of significance in the ongoing participation of T lymphocyte injury.

Besides targeting tumor antigens and inducing tumor cell death, tumor antigen-targeting monoclonal antibodies interact with immune cells through Fc-dependent mechanisms to induce adaptive memory immune responses [9].

IMMUNE TOLERANCE

The significance of immune tolerance is further projected by models of tumor progression within the system profiles of induction, and also non-induction, of pathways of metabolic co-operativity. In such terms, ongoing events incorporate the proposed pathway nomogram as induced by intermediates of such pathways. The induction of actual dimensions are contextual conformity within systems of response, and also nonresponse, to tumor neoantigenicity. The magnitude and the type of immune response depends on the local cytokine milieu and the aryl hydrocarbon receptor is one key factor involved in the fine-tuning of this cytokine balance [10].

In terms that bespeak of such inducive actions, the property realization of T lymphocyte response is cardinal consideration within systems as projected within frameworks for further development of immune tolerance to tumor neoantigenicity.

CONCLUSION

The conclusive phenomena that contribute to a sustained immunologic tolerance are derivative metabolite system series that incorporate the compound profiles for further generation of immune suppression. IDO is over expressed in both cancer cells and antigen-presenting cells in tumor-draining lymph nodes where it promotes peripheral immune tolerance to tumor antigens; inhibitors of IDO reverse this immunosuppression, complementing classical cytotoxic cancer chemotherapy [11]. In such terms, the contextual cellular contact events are also persistent inducing series of influences that partake as further phenomena of sustainment biology mechanics. The proposed incorporation of antigenicity as foreign elements is well exemplified by the infectious and parasitic dimensions of such antigen exposure.

In the case of tumors, the co-operative performance of dimensionality is proposed sustainment of such antigen exposure as provided by pathway metabolic events. The proposed significance of such phenomena is inducing influence per se as proposed by tumor antigenicity. Further idealization formulas are pathway-derived within the compounding effects of events primarily of antigenicity-suppressive action in generating tolerogenicity.

References

[1] Santoiemma PP, Powell DJ Jr "Tumor infiltrating lymphocytes in ovarian cancer" *Cancer Biol There* 2015;16(6):807-20.

[2] Pockley AG, Vaupel P, Multhoff G "NK cell-based therapeutics for lung cancer" *Expert Opin Biol There* 2020;30(1):23-33.

[3] Liu M, Li Ziyang, Yao W, Zeng X, Wang L, Cheng J et al "IDO inhibitor synergised with radiotherapy to delay tumor growth by reversing T cell exhaustion" *Mol Med Rep* 2020;21(1):445-453.

[4] Chen X, Pan X, Zhang W, Guo H, Cheng S, He Q et al. "Epigenetic strategies synergies with PD-L1/PD-1 targeted cancer immunotherapies to enhance antitumor responses" *Acta Pharm Sin B* 2020;10(5):723-733.

[5] Lu J, Liu X, Liao YP, Wang X, Ahmed A, Jiang W et al. "Breast cancer chemo-immunotherapy through liposomal delivery of an immunogenic cell death stimulus plus interference in the IDO-1 pathway" *ACS Nano* 2018;12(11):11041-11061.

[6] Le Naour J, Galluzzi L, Zitvogel L, Kroemer G, Vacchelli E "Trial watch: IDO inhibitors in cancer therapy" *Oncoimmunology* 2020;9(1):1777625.

[7] Popov A, Schultze JL "IDO-expressing regulatory dendritic cells in cancer and chronic infection" *J Mol Med* (Berl) 2008;86(2):145-60.

[8] Liu X, Shin N, Koblish HK, Yang G, Wang Q, Wang K et al. "Selective inhibition of IDO1 effectively regulates mediators of antitumor immunity" *Blood* 2019;115(17):3520-30.

[9] Michaud HA, Eliaou JF, Lafont V, Bonnefoy N, Gros L "Tumor antigen-targeting monoclonal antibody-based immunotherapy: orchestrating combined strategies for the development of long-term antitumor immunity" *Oncoimmunology* 2014;3(9):e955684.

[10] Hao N, Whitelaw ML "The emerging roles of AhR in physiology and immunity" *Biochem Pharmacy* 2013;86(5):561-70.

[11] Katz JB, Muller AJ, Prendergast GC "Indoleamine 2,3-dioxygenase in T-cell tolerance and tumor immune escape" *Immune Rev* 2008;222:206-21.

Chapter 5

INCONGRUENT BIOLOGY OF REDISTRIBUTED CHEMOKINE ACTION IN CARCINOGENESIS

ABSTRACT

The promotional antigenicity profiles exhibited by proliferating tumor cells allows for a permissive microenvironment as projected by immature DC. It is within redefined milieu of chemokine reactivity that redistribution of antigenic stimuli allow for projected modulations of the integral immune systems as proposed by the redefined chemokine reactivity. It is the simple juxtaposition of multiple range of antigenicity that perforce allows for immune tolerance and permissiveness to emerge. The recharacterization of such antigenicity is recharacterization of inherent component pathway reactivity as indeed projected chemokine redistribution within profiles of the immune response to proliferating tumor cell beds.

INTRODUCTION

The distributional functionality of dendritic cells (DC) is an integral reflection of the constitutive determination of a potent anti-tumoral immunity within the scope of participation of tumor-related dysfunction of reactivity. Macrophages infiltrating tumors are driven by tumor-derived and T cell-derived cytokines to acquire a polarised M2 phenotype [1]. It is within such scope of involvement, as manifested in the sentinel lymph node, that the incongruity of immune response to tumor antigenicity allows for a permissive microenvironment, within the encompassed derivative of tumor cell secretion of immunosuppressive molecules. Intra-tumoral Batf3 DC are necessary for effector T cell trafficking and adoptive T cell therapy [2]. In such terms, the ongoing derivation of tumor cells and of their induced dysfunction allows for the emergence of pathway reactivity as mediated by immature DC, and as further proposed by dimensions of intricate complexity as denoted by varying degree of immaturity of the DC. CCL18 is a marker of the M2 macrophages and an increased production of CCL18 is related to the immunosuppressive nature of the tumor microenvironment [3].

It is within such scenario of nonreactivity that the dimensions of chemokine secretion permits the realization of tumor-cell injury as further propounded pathways for further immunosuppression.

Distributional Biology

The distributional anatomy and functionality of suppressive T cells constitutes the emergence of processed antigen by mature and immature DC, as further exhibited within confines for further immunosuppression. NK cells enhance recruitment of conventional DC1 into the tumor microenvironment promoting immune control of the cancer lesion [4]. The realization of tumor-cell induced suppression allows for a redefinition of permissive microenvironment, as indeed proposed by pathway incongruity and as further proposed by substantial involvement of pattern recognition pathways induced by tumor cell antigenicity. Heterodimeric IL-15 delays cancer growth and enhances intratumoral CTL and dendritic cell accumulation by a cytokine network including XCL1, IFN-gamma, CXCL9 and CXCL10 [5, 6].

CCL20 signaling is also implicated in the tumor microenvironment and contributes to cancer progression as in liver and colon cancer, breast and pancreatic cancer and in gastric cancer [7]. It is in the realization of such injury to tumor cells that a whole panorama of dimensional redistribution of DC allows for the generation of regulatory T cells, and for the dysfunction induced by indoleamine 2,3 dioxygenase-bearing immune cells.

Confined Attribute Dysfunction

In terms attributable within encompassed confinement of attribute dysfunction of the immune system that there evolves the dimensionality of incongruence of antigen presentation by mature DC. It is the range of distributional dysfunctionality that the whole process of immunosuppression is instituted within system pathways of recognition at the earliest stages of determination of tumor-cell antigenicity. The cooperation between tumor-derived CCL5 and IFN-gamma-inducible CXCR3 ligands produced by myeloid cells is central for orchestrating T cell infiltration in immunoreactive and immunoresponsive cancers [8].

It is within the confinement of such antigenicity that ongoing pathways of reactivity allow for permissive microenvironments, as borne out by systems of pattern molecules released during tumor-cell injury.

Dimensionality

Systems of proposed dimensionality include the proponent chemoreactivity that recontributes to a chemokine-induced series of wave dysfunctions in response to tumor-cell reactivity. The pathway component biology is further conformational redistribution as borne out by the dynamics of incongruity by tumor-cell injury. CCL14 expression in hepatocellular cancer correlates with exhausted Tcell markers, PD-1, TIM-3 and CTLA-4, suggesting a role in regulating tumor immunity [9].

Cross-priming in which DC activate CD8 T cells by cross-presenting exogenous antigens is critical in generating anti-tumor CD8 T cell immunity [10].

Multiple pathways for such recognition of tumor-cell antigenicity allows for redefinition of systems of patterned molecular recognition, as indeed outlined by the component realization of permissive microenvironment inherent to a generic dimension of proposed tumor-cell injury and antigenicity. CD103 integrin triggers bidirectional signaling events that cooperate with TCR signals to potentiate T-cell migration and optimal cytokine production [11].

Immaturity of Dendritic Cells

Proposed redistribution of DC and of primed T lymphocytes is cardinal proposition within further conformational biology of cell interactivity within the outlined emergence of cytotoxic and helper T cells. Peripheral CD103+ DC form a unified subset developmentally allied to CD8alpha+ conventional DC [12]. Hence transport mechanics for redistribution of primed T cells is component realization, as further emergent components for further activation of DC and lymphocytes.

In such terms, the emergent recapitulation of primed T cells allows for the marker status of primed T cells within systems of recognition of antigen at very early stages of instituted tumor-cell antigenicity.

Beyond simple dimensions of antigenicity, the proponent permissiveness of tumor cell antigenicity proposes the modulated microenvironment as projected within the intratumoral and peritumoral microenvironment. Hypoxia alters the expression of CC chemokine and CC chemokine receptors in tumors [13]. The realization of regulatory DC, and of immaturity of such DC, propagates a redistributional dysfunction as evidenced by pathway nonresolution. Many studies have confirmed that chemokine receptor 9 and its exclusive ligand chemokine

25 are over-expressed in many types of cancer and are closely related to tumor proliferation, apoptosis, invasion, migration and drug resistance [14].

MOLECULAR PATTERNS OF RECOGNITION

Patterns of molecular recognition are targeted dynamics for non-resolution of the tumor cell antigenicity, as confined proposition within systems for redistribution of the antigenic molecules, as projected by a permissive and immune suppression. Component incongruity is derived projection for abnormal redistribution of antigenic stimuli, as terms for further tumor-cell proliferation and spread. The proposed machinery for modulated tumor-cell antigenicity is inherent characterized and recharacterized dimensions as terms of patterned molecular recognition by the DC. The derivative dimensions for such tumor cell antigenicity is compound nonresolution within terms of reference of chemokine dynamics.

PATHWAY NONRESOLUTION

Pathway nonresolution is molecularly redefined, as indeed proposed by redistribution of antigen-loaded DC, and as outlined by the incongruity of emergent tumor cell antigenicity.

Regulatory T cells and DC are response pathway definitions, as terms projected by incongruent nonrecognition of the tumor cell antigenicity, and as further proposed by dimensions of reconstituted homeostasis of immune dynamics. Such incongruence is itself a patterned redistribution as carried forward by immature and regulatory DC. The conformational redefinition of targeted dynamics of such DC is component biology inherent within an immune responsiveness. The component reappraisal mechanics allows for a failure in reconstitutive response by the integral immune system as a whole. The promotional disproportion of system pathways is hence a pattern recognition of chemokine molecules within early stage dynamics of the emergent tumor cells. Chemotactic cytokines regulate the migration, positioning and interaction of various cell subsets with both anti- and pro-tumor functionality [15]. The incumbent disproportion allows for multiple redefinitions of tumor-cell antigenicity, as further proposed by dynamics of turnover of DC and of primed T lymphocytes.

CONCLUSION

Compound chemokine dynamics develop as redistributionally redefined tumor cell antigenicity as carried forward by the emergence of immature and regulatory DC. The performance dynamics of an antitumor reactivity propounds the projected targets of tumor antigens as further involved redistribution of such antigenicity. The dimensional recharacterization of antigenicity proposes a revised profile for parameters of targeting immunity that further evolves as permissive elements of reconstitution of quasi homeostasis. The performance of the antigen targeting is incumbent of the pathway reactivities of the immune system as a whole and within confined redistribution of chemokine action. The simple recognition of patterns of antigenicity are re-dimensionalized within the profile biology of an antigen series of responses as proposed by highly proliferative and spreading tumor-cell beds. In such terms, incongruent recognition of antigens is an innate immune response of pathway non-recognition at early stages of carcinogenesis.

REFERENCES

[1] Mantovani A, Sozzani S, Locati M, Allavena P, Sica A "Macrophage polarisation: tumor-associated macrophages as a paradigm for polarised M2 mononuclear phagocytes" *Trends Immunol* 2002;23(11):549-55.

[2] Spranger S, Dai D, Horton B, Gajewski TF "Tumor-residing Batf3 dendritic cells are required for effector T cell trafficking and adoptive T cell therapy" *Cancer Cell* 2017;31(5):711-723.

[3] Korbecki J, Olbromski M, Dziegiel P "CCL18 in the progression of cancer" *Int J Mol Sci* 2020;21(21):7955.

[4] Bottcher JP, Bonavita E, Chakravarty P, Blees H, Cabeza-Cabrerizo M, Sammicheli S et al. "NK cells stimulate recruitment of cDC1 into the tumor microenvironment promoting cancer immune control" *Cell* 2018;172(5):1022-1037.

[5] Bergamaschi C, Pandit H, Nagy BA, Stellas D, Jensen SM, Bear J et al. "Heterodimeric IL-15 delays tumor growth and promotes intratumoral CTL and dendritic cell accumulation by a cytokine network involving XCL1, IFN-gamma, CXCL9 and CXCL10" *J Immunother Cancer* 2020;8(1):e000599.

[6] Korbecki J, Grochans S, Gutowska I, Barczak K, Baranowska-Bosiacka I "CC chemokines in a tumor: a review of pro-cancer and anti-cancer properties of receptors CCR5, CCR6, CCR7, CCR8, CCR9, and CCR10 ligands" *Int J Mol Sci* 2020;21(20):7619.

[7] Chen W, Qin Y, Liu S "CCL20 signaling in the tumor microenvironment" *Adv Exp Med Biol* 2020;1231:53-65.

[8] Dangaj D, Bruand M, Grimm AJ, Ronet C, Barras D, Duttagupta PA et al. "Cooperation between constitutive and inducible chemokine enables T cell engraftment and immune attack in solid tumors" *Cancer Cell* 2019;35(6):885-900.

[9] Gu Y, Li X, Bi Y, Zheng Y, Wang J, Li X et al. "CCL14 is a prognostic biomarker and correlates with immune infiltrates in hepatocellular carcinoma" *Aging* (Albany NY) 2020;12(1):784-807. 60.

[10] Fu C, Jiang A "Dendritic cells and CD8 T cell immunity in tumor microenvironment" *Front Immunol* 2018;9:3059.

[11] Corgnac S, Boutet M, Kfoury M, Naltet C, Mami-Chouaib F "The emerging role of CD8+ tissue resident memory T (T rm) cells in antitumor immunity: a unique functional contribution of the CD103 integrin" *Front Immunol* 2018;9:1904.

[12] Edelson BT, KC W, Juang R, Kohyama M, Benoit LA, Klekotka PA et al. "Peripheral CD103+ dendritic cells form a unified subset developmentally related to CD8alpha+ conventional dendritic cells" *J Exp Med* 2010;207(4):823-36.

[13] Korbecki J, Kojder K, Barczak K, Siminska D, Gutowska I, Chlubek D et al. "Hypoxia alters the expression of CC chemokine and CC chemokine receptors in a tumor—a literature review" *Int J Mol Sci* 2020;21(16):5647.

[14] Xu B, Deng C, Wu X, Ji T, Zhao L, Han Y et al. "CCR9 and CCL25: a review of their roles in tumor promotion" *J Cell Physiol* 2020;235(12):9121-9132.

[15] Cardoso AP, Pinto ML, Castro F, Costa AM, Marques-Magalhaes A, Canha-Borges A et al. "The immunosuppressive and pro-tumor functions of CCL18 at the tutor microenvironment" *Cytokine Growth Factor Rev* 2021;60:107-119.

Chapter 6

THE NATURE OF MODULATED REDISTRIBUTION OF INTEGRAL IMMUNITY AS SYSTEM REDEFINITION OF CLINICAL NON-RESPONSIVENESS TO THE ANTITUMOR ANTIGENICITY

ABSTRACT

The dynamics of the evolving antitumor immune response arise as a primal attribute of a generic induction phenomenon originating in terms of antigen presentation by dendritic cells. The integrated nature of the innate and adaptive immune systems is performance dynamics of a conceptual series of system pathways that evolve primarily and exclusively as dynamics of modulation pathways that incorporate the regulatory control of immune responsiveness. The particular dynamics of evolution of immune responses are therefore re-characterizations of the prominent role of antigen presentation by dendritic cells in conformation to the redistributed participation of immunosuppressants and immunostimulatory effects of response.

INTRODUCTON

The similitude of vaccination procedures incorporates a series of stimulatory events within the scope of multiple participants that induce generic processes in immune response, including the diversity of dendritic cell (DC) -based procedures in attempted antitumor effect, Trained immune training of granulopoiesis through the modulation of mature myeloid cells or their bone marrow progenitors, induces sustained responsiveness to anti-tumor activity [1]. In terms of an ongoing participation of immune system targeting, it is significant to view the diversity of modes of approach as particular specificities that evolve primarily as generic induction. The development of cancer vaccines has proved slow with limited clinical efficacy [2]. The particular dimensions of incorporation of immune responses are hence primarily a series of nonspecific particulars in the setting of CD4+ and CD8+ dimensions that evolve as immune responsiveness, in terms that redefine the significant roles of specific arms of the immune system, including also, and in particular, an incorporation of both adaptive and innate systems.

Cellular and molecular mechanisms of the immune response are essential components of the tumor microenvironment [3]. The participation of various diverse immune responses include the liberated potentialities that respond to the DC-based vaccines that are delivered as stimulants in bolstering antitumor response.

ANTITUMOR IMMUNITY

The specificities of incumbent involvement of the antitumor immune responses are integral to a wide range potentiality that redefines the incorporation of both stimulatory and inhibitory agents, as these are projected within systems for appraisal and re-appraisal by the tumor microenvironment, and as systems for further potential evolution and adaptation. Characterised microenvironment of human tumors has led to the discovery of tertiary lymphoid structures incorporating mature dendritic cells in a T-cell zone adjacent to B-cell follicle including a germinal centre [4].

The realisation of stimulatory antigenicity within the tumor microenvironment allows for a large and diverse series of pre-adaptation phenomena, as carried forward by a multitude of antigenic epitopes presented by the tumor cell populations and by clones of diverse formulations. Several clinical trials utilising immunostimulatory adjuvants, especially agonistic and non-agonistic ligands for Toll-like receptors, C-type lectin receptors, retinoid acid-inducible one 1-like receptors and stimulator of interferon genes, have proved therapeutic not only as vaccine adjuvants but also as antitumor agents [5].

The significant participation of potentiality in antigen presentation is carried forward by a heterogeneous population of dendritic cells (DC) within the tumor cell bed. It is significant to view the various modulators as integral to an involved adaptation of the integrated innate and adaptive immune responsiveness.

The dimensions of incorporation of dimensionality is a particularly radical projection of the integrated immune response that is particularly modified by inhibitory agents for significant suppression of antigenicity, as presented by the incorporated tumor cell population as a whole. Alarming in particular are important as initiators and participants in host defense, regulated gene expression, homeostasis, wound healing, allergy, inflammation, autoimmunity and tumorigenesis [6]. Within the substantial induction by antigenicity, there emerges the diversity of systems of antigen presentation as systems of responsive protection of native antigens carried by normal cells. The "danger" signals created by virus-infected cells appear able to generate immune co-stimulation to override immune suppression and reverse tolerance in the tumor microenvironment [7].

Generic Induction

The generic nature of the antigenicity as presented by DC is carried forward to create immune responses that are largely disassociated with clinical responses to immunotherapies.

In terms, therefore, of a substantial participation of tumor cell injury, the incorporated dimensions of immune responses are significant in terms of an immune system that is primarily suppressed rather than stimulated by native antigenicity. This view of the significant dissociation of the clinical outcome in the face of immune response is the redefinition of potential roles of immune-mediated antigen presentation by DC.

The further participation of generic induction phenomena are pathway specificities within systems of response in terms of system pathway modulation of both innate and adaptive responsiveness. Necroptotic tumor cells release damage-associated molecular patterns and induce maturation of DC, the cross-priming of cytotoxic lymphocytes, and the generation of Interferon-gamma to tumor antigenicity [8].

Substantial incorporation of immune responses are hence obstacles as projected by antitumor involvements of redefined integral immune systems of potential modulation.

Tumors express few neoantigens, and hence are less responsive to immune therapy; new antigens can be induced by transient down regulation of the transporter associated with antigen processing [9]. The nature of evolving immune responsiveness is a significant re-introduction of pathway outlines that involve the well-defined antigenic stimuli that paradoxically redefine the generic nature of induction phenomena in immune responsiveness. The incorporation of integers of suppression of the various arms of the whole immune system responsiveness to tumor antigens is significant as the redefined nature of a system modulation of response that reflects the circumscribed projection of the various forms of immune response.

Pathway Incongruity

Systems of immune response are only partially projected as pathways of evolving influence in modulating tumor antigenicity. Following viral infection of a tumor cell, several events may develop, including direct viral oncolysis, apoptosis, necrotic cell death and autophagic cellular demise [10].

The derived nature of the innate immune system, in particular, is a multi-layered structure that incorporates a large series of modulators that evolve in terms of immune adaptation to the tumor antigenicity. The nature of immune response only partially reflects the ongoing dimensions as natural adaptation to tumor cell antigenicity. Oncolytic measles viruses have been engineered for enhanced antitumor activity, and insertion of immunomodulatory transgenes promotes therapeutic potency [11]. Oncolytic virotherapy is mainly impaired by the host immune response to the viral infection; cytotoxic lymphocytes can induce apoptosis of infected cancer cells and free viruses can be inactivated by neutralising antibodies or cleared by the innate immune response [12].

Immunosuppression

The confounding involvement of immune suppressive agents is a primal pathway of incongruity as carried forward by systems of antigen presentation by the DC. Hence, it is significant to consider the dimensions of antigen presentation as only one facet of the generic induction phenomena induced by tumor antigenicity.

The redefinition of tumor antigens is molecularly compromised in terms of epitope identity and reformulation that are carried forward by the incorporation of action of the immune suppressants in immune responsiveness. The projection of the innate immune system, in particular, is digitalized dimension within systems of pathway culmination and effect. Oncolytic viruses target multiple steps within the cancer-immunity cycle; they can lyse tutor cells, with the generation of soluble antigens, danger signals and type I interferons, in addition to expression of therapeutic genes and as an in situ source of neoantigen vaccination through cross-presentation [13]. The participation of cell injury within tumor cell populations is a reflected non-effectiveness that is carried forward by the identity dynamics for further renewed antigenicity and is further redefined by the modulators of both the innate and adaptive immune responses.

CONCLUSION

The significant aspects of the immune responses to tumor cell antigenicity reflects the incorporated nature of the innate and adaptive immune systems, that are carried forward by conceptual idealisation in pathway incongruity. The significance for evolution of a generic induction phenomenon is integral dimension for responsiveness, as significant re-characterization of the tumor cell antigen presentation process. Dimensional nature of the primal antitumor immune response is a primary consideration of evolving immunity that is only partially reflected in pathway construction and reconstruction.

The existing innate and adaptive immune barriers restricting oncolytic virotherapy, can be overcome using autologous or allogeneic mesenchymal stems c cells in terms of carrier cells with unique abilities for immunosuppression [14].

In view of the participation of tumor cell injury, as incorporated immune responsiveness, the redistribution of antitumor antigen presentation is only a less faithful representation of the dynamics of both the innate and adaptive immune systems in response to growth and spread of the tumor cells. It is highly significant to view the antitumor systems of immune modulation in terms primarily arising in pathway formulations of cause and effect dynamics, and as projected dimensions for the modulated nature of the immune responsiveness to the objective phenomenon of dynamic tumor cell antigen presentation to DC subtypes.

REFERENCES

[1] Kalafati L, Kourtzelis I, Schulte-Schrepping J, Li X, Hatzioannou A, Grinenko T et al. "Innate immune training of granulopoiesis promotes anti-tumor activity" *Cell* 2020;183(3):771-785.

[2] Saliba H, Heurtault B, Bouharoun-Tayoun H, Flacher V, Frisch B, Fournel S et al. "Enhancing tumor specific immune responses by transcutaneous vaccination" *Expert Rev Vaccines* 2017;16(1):1079-1094.

[3] Croci DO, Salatino M "Tumor immune escape mechanisms that operate during metastasis" *Curr Pharm Biotechnol* 2011;12(11):1923-36.

[4] Dieu-Nosjean MC, Giraldo NA, Kaplon H, Germain C, Fridman WH, Sautes-Fridman C "Tertiary lymphoid structures, drivers of the anti-tumor responses in human cancers" *Immunol Rev* 2016;271(1):260-75.

[5] Temizoz B, Kuroda E, Ishii KJ "Vaccine adjuvants as potential cancer immunotherapeutics" *Int Immunol* 2016;28(7):329-38.

[6] Yang D, Han Z, Oppenheim JJ "Alarmins and immunity" *Immunol Rev* 2017;280(1):41-56.

[7] Tong AW, Senzer N, Cerullo V, Templeton NS, Hemminki A, Nemunaitis J "Oncolytic viruses for induction of anti-tumor immunity" *Curr Pharm Biotechnol* 2012;13(9):1750-60.

[8] Aaes TL, Kaczmarek A, Delvaeye T, De Craene B, De Koker S, Heyndrickx L et al. "Vaccination with necroptotic cancer cells induces efficient anti-tumor immunity" *Cell Rep* 2016;15(2):274-87.

[9] Garrido G, Schrand B, Rabasa A, Levay A. D'Eramo F, Berezhnoy A et al. "Tumor-targeted silencing of the peptide transporter TAP induces potent antitumor immunity" *Nat Commun* 2019;10(1):3773.

[10] Atherton MJ, Lichty BD "Evolution of oncolytic viruses: novel strategies for cancer treatment" *Immunotherapy* 2013; 5(11):1191-206.

[11] Grossardt C, England CE, Bossow S, Halama N, Zaoui K, Leber MF et al. "Granulocyte-macrophage colony-stimulating factor-armed oncolytic measles virus is an effective therapeutic cancer vaccine" *Hum Gene There* 2013;24(7):644-54.

[12] Paiva LR, Silva HS, Ferreira SC, Martins ML "Multiscale model for the effects of adaptive immunity suppression on the viral therapy of cancer" *Phys Biol* 2013;10(2):025005.

[13] Bommareddy PK, Shettigar M, Kaufman HL "Integrating oncolytic viruses in combination cancer immunotherapy" *Nat Rev Immunol* 20`8;18(8):498-513.

[14] Draganov DD, Santidrian AF, Minev I, Nguyen D, Kilinc MO, Petrov I et al. "Delivery of oncolytic vaccinia virus by matched allogeneic stem cells overcomes critical innate and adaptive immune barriers" *J Transl Med* 2019;17(1):100.

Chapter 7

COMPLEXITY OF INTER-ACTIVITIES OF SUPPRESSED IMMUNE RESPONSE WITH DENDRITIC CELL DEVELOPMENT AND DIFFERENTIATION IN TUMORS

ABSTRACT

Multiple variable pathways of activation of the immune tolerance state, in response to tumor cell proliferation and spread, are intrinsically linked to induced suppression of the antitumor immune response. Dendritic cells are the major antigen presenting-cell class as relative to the development from myeloid cells in the bone marrow and as distributed pathways in the attempted antitumor consequences of the immune response. Participation dynamics include the derivative de-suppression of such immune tolerance in a manner that includes the shaping of JAK/STAT pathway reactivation of immune tolerance. Hence, immune tolerance is an integral, actively-participant mechanism system in the evolution of a neoplasm that would otherwise be strongly immunogenic.

Complex relative interactions of suppression with activation of the antitumor immune response appear to constitute the emergence dynamics of a series of DNA gene expression profiles that include especially cytokines and growth factors, as well illustrated by the JAK/STAT pathways and by STAT3 in particular. The congruent systems of suppressed and activated DC participation are integral complexes that are realized by immune tolerance in terms of dominant consequences to failed development and differentiation mechanics of the dendritic cells.

INTRODUCTION

The production of soluble factors is major inducer of suppressive effects on dendritic cells (DC) in their stimulation of the antitumor immune response. In such terms, tumor-derived cytokines and growth factors may suppress differentiation and function of DC within an encompassed repertoire of negative dominant effects. It is further to such conditions that JAK/STAT3 suppresses antigen presentation by inducing abnormalities in the DC differentiation pathways.

A relevant proportion of cancer patients does not benefit from immunotherapies ,due partly to an ineffective NK cell activation, a lack of tumor-specific NK cells, an unregulated expression of checkpoint pathways, and a low mutational burden that hinders the emergence of long-term adaptive immunity [1].

PHOSPHORYLATION

The full implications of disrupted maturation of DC is well-illustrated in mice with knockdown of STAT3 gene production and hence is constitutively illustrative of the central role of the STAT3 involvement in suppression of the antitumor immune response. In such terms, ongoing participation of a disrupted or suppressed host immune response against tumors is due, in large measure, to defects of the host immune response. The realization of tumor derived factors arises from the emergence of VEGF, GM CSF, IL-10, IL-6, TGF beta, prostaglandins and gangliosides.

The development of immaturity of DC is therefore a directly induced effect arising in terms of failure of maturation of the antigen-presenting cells due to secretion of tumor-derived soluble factors.

The wide variety of such secreted factors converges, in large measure, on the JAK/STAT3 pathways within simple processes of tyrosine kinase phosphorylation steps. Fibrinogen-like protein 2 is highly expressed in glioma stem cells and primary glioblastoma cells and this is relevant because low levels of this protein factor in association with high granulocyte-colony stimulating factor expression are associated with longer patient survival [2].

Solute carrier transporters regulate lymphocyte signaling and control their differentiation, function and fate by modulating many metabolic pathways and balanced levels of various metabolites; such transporters include glucose transporters, amino-acid transporters, and metal-ion transporters in various pathologic contexts [3].

STAT Dynamics

Docking of STAT proteins on tyrosine residues on the JAK receptor and their DNA binding domain regulates specificity of DNA binding of STAT. SH2 controls interaction with a phosphorylated tyrosine residue at the receptor. STAT dimers translocate to the nucleus to induce specific gene expression.

Activation of STAT3 is also stimulated by acetylation in the C terminal transcriptional activation domain.

Negative regulation of JAK/STAT activity depends on various different mechanisms including phosphatases. Probably, multiple cytokines may be implicated in suppression of DC differentiation. DC development is distinct from DC differentiation and function. Thus, STAT3 may protect against autoimmunity by impaired immune responsiveness to tumors. Hyperphosphorylation of Jak2 leads to activation of STAT3 of hematopoietic cells, critically impairing immature DC differentiation.

Multiple cancer immunotherapies include chimeric antigen receptor T cell and immune checkpoint inhibitors; in addition, the cyclic guanosine monophosphate-adenosine monophosphate synthase—stimulator of interferon genes—TANK-binding kinase is the major signaling pathway for the innate immune response to cancer cells [4].

Ideal Targets

JAK/STAT pathways are ideal targets for enhancing antitumor immune responses and this is supported by pharmacologic inhibition as provided by JSI 124 (cucurbitacin I) by inhibiting cellular levels of phosphotyrosine STAT3 and phospho Jak2. Such action enhances effects of immunotherapy and dramatic activation of immature DC generated in the presence of tumor-derived soluble factors. There is also enhancement of production of pro-inflammatory cytokines such as Interferon-gamma, IL-12, TNF-alpha and IL-2 on combining CpG with JSI 124.

Such considerations indicate the critical need to suppress the JAK/STAT3 pathways in a manner that enhances differentiation of DC. Phosphoryation is a key step in activation of STAT3, supported by acetylation processes. In such measure, the evolutionary dimensions of such constitutive pathways are associated with marked enhancement of DC differentiation, and hence generation of an antitumor immune response.

The gene transcription pathways are associated also with post-translational modifications of proteins in the induction of the antitumor immune reactivities in a manner that is critical to suppression of STAT3 negative regulation of DC differentiation. DC development from hematopoietic cells is also activated, and such enhancement is coupled with a break in the immune tolerance to tumor cells.

In vitro studies show that IL-6-mediated STAT3 activation diminishes surface expression of HLA-DR on CD14+ monocyte-derived DC, with inhibition of functional maturation of DC to stimulate effector T cells [5]. Cyclooxyrgenase 2, arginase and lysosome protease are implicated in IL-6 induced down-regulation of surface expression of HLA class II on human DC.

Evidence suggests that successful anticancer therapy depends on responsiveness of both tumor cells and DC to type I Interferons [6].

COMPLEXITY

The linkage of the distinct pathways of DC development, on the one hand, with DC differentiation mirror the different mechanistic pathways, in complex fashion, towards an antitumor immune response that is augmented within systems of persistent suppression of tumor cell growth and spread. In such manner, the evolutionary dimensions for further control of JAK/STAT pathways constitute the mechanistic stimulation for activation of the antitumor immune response. Understanding the molecular modulation of neutrophils, macrophages, and DC is required to develop novel approaches to treat cancer and autoimmunity [7].

CONCLUSION

A general concept of de-suppression effects on the JAK/STAT pathways is a mechanistically illustrative example that is carried forward by the dominant roles of tumor-secreted soluble factors that otherwise induce immune tolerance. In such terms, the incremental dimensions of tumor growth and spread are integral constitutive measures in the formulation of a failed immune response, in spite of the neoantigenicity of tumor cells.

The emergence of trafficking of DC to and within secondary lymphoid organs, and the activation of the immune response, are participant factors in conformation with the initial development of DC from hematopoietic progenitor cells and the subsequent differentiation of activated DC.

In terms beyond simple activation of an antitumor immune response, the milieu of the tumor microenvironment also includes macrophages associated with the tumor in the first instance. It is significant to view the liability of generation of neoplastic cells that develop as carcinogenetic product of the suppressed DC development and of impaired DC differentiation, beyond the activation steps in immune responsiveness. STAT1 and STAT3 are utilised by cytokines to modulate the signal output of heterologous receptors of the innate immune response, including pattern recognition receptors and affecting also oncogenic and metabolic cell processes [8]. Cytokines activate the Janus Kinases and STAT members to modulate lymphoid development and sustain T-cell activation and differentiation [9].

The emergence of contingent factors secreted by tumors may constitute further targeting opportunities within simple de-suppression of the JAK/STAT pathways, and within simple recognizable systems of suppression of the immune response.

REFERENCES

[1] Pockley AG, Vaupel P, Multhoff G "NK cell-based therapeutics for lung cancer" *Expert Opin Biol There* 2020;20(1):23-33.

[2] Yan J, Zhao Q, Gabrusiewicz K, Kong LY, Xia X, Wang J et al. "FGL2 promotes tumor progression in the CNS by suppressing CD103(+) dendritic cell differentiation" *Nat Commun* 2019;10(1):448.

[3] Song W, Li D. Tao L, Luo Q, Chen L "Solute carrier transporters: the metabolic gatekeepers of immune cells" *Acta Pharm Sin B* 2020;10(1):61-78.

[4] Ding C, Song Z, Shen A, Chen T, Zhang A "Small molecules targeting the innate immune cGAS-STING-TBK1 signaling pathway" *Acta Pharm Sin B* 2020;10(12):2272-2298.

[5] Kitamura H, Ohno Y, Toyoshima Y, Ohtake J, Homma S, Kawamura H et al. "Interleukin-6/STAT3 signaling as a promising

target to improve the efficacy of cancer immunotherapy" *Cancer Sci* 2017;108(10):1947-1952.

[6] Sprooten J, Agostinis P, Garg AD "Type I interferons and dendritic cells in cancer immunotherapy" *Int Rev Cell Mol Biol* 2019;348:217-262.

[7] Li HS, Watowich SS "Innate immune regulation by STAT-mediated transcriptional mechanisms" *Immunol Rev* 2014;261(1):84-101.

[8] Jenkins BJ "Transcriptional regulation of pattern recognition receptors by Jak/STAT signaling, and the implications for disease pathogenesis" *J Interferon Cytokine Res* 2014;34(10):750-8.

[9] Stabile H, Scarno G, Fionda C, Gismondi A, Santoni A, Gadina M et al. "JAK/STAT signaling in regulation of innate lymphoid cells: the gods before the guardians" *Immunol Rev* 2018;286(1):148-159.

Chapter 8

System Profiles of Dendritic Cell Motility as Modeled Tumor Cell Proliferation and Spread

Abstract

Models of the immune response recaptulate the significant degree of mobility of DC within profiles for redistribution of antigenicity as provoked by the further conformations of a constitutive modality interactivity between DC and tumor cells. In such scenario, the further projection of motility and spread of DC is a confirmatory reappraisal of the biologic and pathobiologic mechanics of tumor cell proliferation and spread within system dimensions for further tumor growth. In such terms of a constitutive attribute of immune tolerance to tumor antigenicity there emerges a concept for inherent modulation of DC as dominated by tumor antigenicity as a generic property of malignant transformation.

Introduction

Constitutive activation of dendritic cells (DC) allows an inherent susceptibility to the emergence of tolerogenic subsets of DC within a system profile of further suppression of the immune response. In such terms, the ongoing stimulation of immunologic competence is beset by the development of soluble cell-derived factors that the tumor and microenvironment provoke within such systems, promoting DC plasticity.

Natural killer cells can limit or exacerbate immune responses; they limit tumor spread and subsequent tissue damage [1].

The promotion of the immune response to tumors in particular constitute the recharacterization and skewing of the DC within the susceptibility profile as presented by a series of events that tend to modulate the tumor microenvironment as presented to DC. Tissue-resident memory CD8+ T cells propagate antitumor immunity by triggering antigen spreading via dendritic cells [2].

It is particularly significant that incorporation of avoidance pathways to the immune response largely concerns dendritic cell presentation of tumor antigen and would further exacerbate DC plasticity. Aberrant over expression and glycosylation of mucins in various malignant neoplasms facilitate oncogenic events from inception to spread [3].

PERFORMANCE CRITERIA

The performance criteria of DC antigen presentation appear to promote the emergence of an integral DC antigenicity in its own right within the system mirroring capacity for further antigen presentation. Augmenting endogenous DC is a promising strategy to overcome antigen-negative tumor escape following adoptive cell treatment (4). In such terms, the provocative redistribution of DC is constitutively progressive as well attested by migratory performance of the DC. Suboptimal patient outcome is probably due in part to the complex network of immunosuppressive pathways in advanced neoplasms [5].

System profile redistribution of DC is system profile modeling that enhances antigen presentation to a wide variety of cells as shown by the evolving plasticity of DC. Loss of galectin-9 expression is closely associated with metastatic progression [6]. The prevocational roles as indeed exhibited by antigen-presenting cells are therefore the motility potential that is promoted by immune response kinetics. In such terms, the actual initial emergence of tumor antigenicity is reflected in highly faithful fashion to a DC module for further skewing of the antigen presenting DC. It is highly significant to view DC performance as an inherent attribute paradoxically arising within systems of progressive tolerance mechanics.

SYSTEM PROFILES

System profile dynamics are thus the promotional performance attributes that inherently comprise stress induction as related not only to tumor cell proliferation and spread but also to treatment induced modulation of the tumor microenvironment.

Cell death induced by CD8+ T cells is immunogenic and primes caspase-3 dependent spread immunity against neoplasm antigens [7]. It is beyond such considerations of DC modulation that the profile management of susceptibility issues of the tumor cell dynamics that there evolves the conspicuous parameters for further proliferation and spread of the tumor cells. Native or genetically modified viruses with oncolytic activity can increase anti-tumor activity in responses to the release of new antigens and danger signals as a result of infection and tumor cell lysis [8].

PLASTICITY OF DC

Plasticity modulation of DC is hence a priority issue in the evolving immune tolerance to tumor growth and spread as faithfully projected within system models of the potentially wide-ranging of the immune response to tumors. In clearly defined projects for further tumor growth and spread the distinctive formulation of injury profiles induced by tumors is stress-provoked and sustained as such.

In such terms, provocative redistribution of DC is reflected in highly constitutive plasticity of immune responses.

System preference of interactivity of DC is hence a mobility attribute of such cells as further attested by the promotional redistribution of immune responsive cells within such organs as regional lymph nodes, spleen and thymus medulla. It is significant to reappraise the immune response as a highly constitutive attribute of such DC motility and mobility within the tumor microenvironment and also as systemic spread. As such, the spread of malignant tumor cells is reflected in a highly faithful manner in the inherent tendency and potential progression of tumor cell proliferation and spread. An ongoing cytotoxic antitumor immune response can provoke immunogenic tumor cell death [9].

MODELED PROFILES

System profile models relate analogously to the biologic attributes of macrophages in general and bespeak of a constitutive tendency to provoke a high variety of cytokine secretion and action.

Both replication-competent and replication-deficient herpes simplex virus 1 may serve as vaccine vectors, and thus tumor regression by stimulation of plasmacytoid dendritic cells [10]. Oncolytic viruses preferentially replicate in neoplasms as compared to normal tissue and enhance immunogenic cell death and induction of host systemic antitumor immunity [11].

The redistribution dynamics of DC are hence module induction of tumor cell proliferation and spread as attested by the convergent integrity of the immune response to tumor cell antigenicity. In such terms, the significant skewing of the DC is further provoked by the system models of an immune response that is primarily tolerogenic and only secondarily reactive. Such a concept of modulated immune response hence arises within profile dynamics projected as immune tolerance.

Robust anti-tumor immunity necessitates innate as well as adaptive immune response [12].

The tumoricidal effect of plasmacytoid dendritic cells and their capacity to overcome the immunosuppressive tumor microenvironment are being investigated [13].

Promotional DC mobility hence is a further testimony to the varied potentials of tumor cell induced response within the profile management for further proliferation and spread of the neoplastic cells. The performance of the immune response in the initial event of tumorigenesis is symptomatic for the realized tolerance of the immune response in terms further promoting redistribution mechanics of both DC and malignant tumor cells. In a realized dynamics of cellular spread and redistribution there therefore emerges the system profile of strict performance templates as assigned to tumor cell turnover.

Genetic engineering of oncolytic viruses have provided improved specificity ad efficacy of oncolytic viruses in cancer treatment [14].

CONCLUSION

Templates of performance dynamics of tumor cell proliferation and spread are applicable to a highly motile population of regional and system subsets of DC within profile mirroring inducive to DC motility and performance. In such terms, the significant reference for tumor biologic activities are paramount considerations in the emergence of immune tolerance as centered on DC performance in the tumor microenvironment. The emergence of dynamic interaction would indicate the template profiles of DC turnover as incumbent attribute of the immune response. The further defining terms of modeled performance hence attribute a realization as projected within systems of DC subset profiles that persistently modulate a whole series of modeled immune responses.

REFERENCES

[1] Vivier E, Tomasello E, Baratin M, Walzer T, Ugolini S "Functions of natural killer cells" *Nat Immunol* 2008;9(5):503-10.

[2] Menares E, Galvez-Cancino F, Caceres-Morgado P, Ghorani E, Lopez E, Diaz X et al." Tissue-resident memory CD8+ T cells amplify anti-tumor immunity by triggering antigen spreading through dendritic cells" *Nat Commun* 2019;10(1):4401.

[3] Bhati R, Gautam SK, Cannon A, Thompson C, Hall BR, Aithal A et al. "Cancer-associated mucins: role in immune modulation and metastasis" *Cancer Metastasis Rev* 2019;38(1-2):223-236.

[4] Lai J, Mardiana S, House IG, Sek K, Henderson MA, Giuffrida L, Chen AXY et al. "Adoptive cellular therapy with T cells expressing the dendritic cell growth factor Flt3L drives epitope spreading and antitumor immunity" *Nat Immunol* 2020:21(8):914-926.

[5] Moynihan KD, Opel CF, Szeto GL, Tzeng A, Zhu EF, Engreitz JM et al. "Eradication of large established tumors in mice by combination immunotherapy that engages innate and adaptive immune responses" *Nat Med* 2016;22(12):1402-1410.

[6] Fujihara S, Mori H, Kobara H, Rafiq K, Niki T, Hiroshima M et al. "Galectin-9 in cancer therapy" *Recent Pat Endocr Metab Immune Drug Discov* 2013;7(2):130-7.

[7] Jaime-Sanchez P, Uranga-Murillo I, Aguilo N, Khouili SC, Arias MA, Sancho D et al. "Cell death induced by cytotoxic CD8(+) T cells is immunogenic and primes caspase-3-dependent spread immunity against endogenous tumor antigens" *J Immunother Cancer* 2020;8(1):e000528.

[8] Marin-Acevedo JA, Soyano AE, Dholaria B, Knutson KL, Lou Y "Cancer immunotherapy beyond immune checkpoint inhibitors" *J Hematol Oncol* 2018;11(1):8.

[9] Minute L, Teijeira A, Sanchez-Paulete AR, Ochoa MC, Alvarez M et al. "Cellular cytotoxicity is a form of immunogenic cell death" *J Immunother Cancer* 2020;8(1):e000325.

[10] Schuster P, Lindner G, Thomann S, Haferkamp S, Schmidt B "Prospect of plasmacytoid dendritic cells in enhancing anti-tumor immunity of oncolytic herpes viruses" *Cancers* (Basel)2019;11(5):651.

[11] Thomas S, Kuncheria L, Roulstone V, Kyula JN, Mansfield D, Bommareddy PK et al. "Development of a new fusion-enhanced oncolytic immunotherapy platform based on herpes simplex virus type 1" *J Immunother Cancer* 2019;7(1):214.

[12] Boscheinen JB, Thomann S, Knipe DM, DeLuca N, Schuler-Thurner B, Gross S et al. "Generation of an oncolytic herpes simplex virus 1 expressing human MelanA" *Front Immune* 2019;10:2.

[13] Thomann S, Boscheinen JB, Vogel K, Knipe DM, DeLuca N, Gross S et al. "Combined cytotoxic activity of an infectious, but non-replicative herpes simplex virus type 1 and plasmacytoid dendritic cells against tumor cells" *Immunology* 2015;146(2):327-38.

[14] Sanchala DS, Bhatt LK, Prabhavalkar KS "Oncolytic herpes simplex viral therapy: a stride toward selective targeting of cancer cells" *Front Pharmacy* 2017;8:270.

Chapter 9

DUALITY OF UNSTABLE DYNAMICS OF EMERGING TUMOR CELLS AND OF INFILTRATING DENDRITIC CELLS IN CARCINOGENESIS

ABSTRACT

Evolving dynamics of instability of antigenicity of tumor cells are closely associated with the emergence of infiltration of the tumor cells by dendritic cells that to a greater or lesser extent involve cellular interactions and antigen presentation to the immune system. The added complexity is conformational paradigm within the evolution of the essential instability phenomena that redefine the system profiles of tumor cell proliferation and spread. In terms therefore of unique antigenicity profiles the essential complexity of system definition as projected by the innate and adaptive immune systems proposes an interactivity within the immune system responses that beset the evolutionary history of a given neoplastic lesion.

INTRODUCTION

The contrasting dynamics of immature versus mature dendritic cells (DC) is a paramount consideration in the analysis of the density and local distribution of these cells in various types of organ neoplasms. Tumor vaccines targeting neoantigens mainly include nucleic acid, dendritic cell-based, tumor cell, and synthetic long peptide vaccines; the prediction of neoantigen affinity to major histocompatibility complexes or the immunogenicity of neoantigens mainly involve whole-exome sequencing technology [1]. It is significant to consider immature DC as an effective index of the potential for differentiation and maturation of this heterogeneous subset of leukocytes derived from hematopoietic bone marrow progenitors. In terms, therefore, of the partly controversial reports of DC, there evolves a highly differential process of evolution of specific different histopathologic types of neoplasms.

TUMOR LESIONS

Melanoma tumor cells are derivative neoplasms that are often aggressive biologic types of tumors that progress continuously with the development of metastatic deposits. Yet, rarely, well documented cases of spontaneous regression of melanoma are reported, indeed in spite of the quasi uniformly aggressive behavior in most patients.

Such a phenomenon is suggestive of a relative relevance of biologic tumor aggressiveness with the rare spontaneity of the tumor regression. Programmed cell death protein 1 plays an important role in eliciting the immune checkpoint response of T cells with consequent evasion of immune surveillance and also refractoriness to conventional chemotherapy [2]. In such terms, the ongoing spread of the tumor may be linked to the differential density of DC within the tumor cell nests or in the intervening stroma of the tumor. In addition to initiating potent anti-tumor immune responses, DC may induce genomic injury, support neovascularization, block anti-tumor immunity and enhance cancerous cell growth and spread [3].

Indeed, ongoing investigations indicate a lymphocytic infiltrate as this regressing tumor subtype proceeds with the added evidence for possible maturation of the DC.

COMPLEXITY OF INTERACTION

The complexity of the distribution of DC within the skin has prevented the full elucidation of the dynamics of turnover of DC within the cutaneous development of a melanoma. The realization of cell injury to such environmental agents as ultraviolet light exposure to the skin indicates the complexity and balancing patterns of various carcinogenic phenomena in the causation of this tumor subset.

Distributional irrelevance of melanoma affliction within the local microenvironment of the occurring early melanoma lesion is promoting consideration within systems that are dynamically unstable. Patients with rare mismatch repair deficiency or micro satellite instability have exquisite sensitivity to checkpoint inhibition in cancer [4]. In such terms, evolving factors in modulation of carcinogenesis negates a well-defined series of differentiation and maturation within the emerging tumor cells themselves.

MicroRNA-21 increases the levels of IL-10 and prostaglandin E2, which inhibit antitumor T-cell-mediated adaptive immunity through suppression of antigen-presentation by DC and T-cell proliferation in colorectal tumors [5].

NON-PATTERN DIFFERENTIATION

Considering the pattern differentiation of DC infiltrating a particular tumor lesion, there is needed a better delineation of the differentiation patterns of the tumor cells themselves within the encompassed derivation from cutaneous melanocytes in the affected skin region. Diverse immune checkpoint inhibitors are being applied for the treatment of melanoma, kidney cancer, lung cancer and also tutors with micro satellite instability [6]. Integration of tutor molecular profiling in trials exploring targeted immunotherapy promote understanding of the predictive role of various molecular and immune biomarkers [7].

It is highly significant to view tumors that from very early origin are dynamically unstable, and also unstable as results of the particular carcinogenic events initiating tumorigenesis.

Chemotherapy-induced ileal crypt apoptosis and the ideal micro biome determine immunosurveillance and progress in patients with proximal colon cancer [8]. In terms indeed of a cyclical process of repeated redefinition of the DC infiltrating the early lesion the process of early carcinogenesis has to be redefined within system profiles of depletion of the DC as viewed by such laboratory investigations as immunohistochemistry and in situ hybridization. Impairments in the immune cycle can be restored by epigenetic modification, including reprogramming the environment of tumor-associated immunity, eliciting an immune response through enhanced tumor antigen presentation and by regulating T cell trafficking and reactivation [9].

MATURATION INDEX

There appears to be a tightly coupled association of the maturation density of DC and the differentiation of the tumor cells in the early stages of carcinogenesis with the added improviso of an escalating cascade series of events as the unstable neoplastic cells become established within the local microenvironment of the involved lesion.

The evolutionary history of a tumor lesion is beset by dynamics of reconstitutive events as provided by such factors as the relation of the immature DC that in their own right evolve also.

In such terms, a duality of involvement of the system profiles of unstable tumor cells emerges within the context provided by infiltrating DC. It is further to such considerations that DC are potent antigen-processing and antigen presenting cells as derived within systems of redefinition of the tumor antigens themselves. It is therefore relevant to consider the individuality of specific subtypes of tumor within the context of individuality of the infiltrating DC within these tumors. The combination of CD8+ T-cell tumor infiltrating lymphocytes, PD-L1 expression, and tumor mutation burden is associated with reliable prognosis [10]. The relevance of intricate interaction also evolves as an index of instability that permits the incorporation of novel neoantigenicity as provided by carcinogenesis.

Clinical Import

Much of the clinical relevance and import of the tumorigenesis phenomenon is linked closely to the emergence of instability in tumor initiation and progression. The relevance of system instability is beset by the attempts to recategorize carcinogenesis within subset tumor categories.

Ligand binding to inhibitory receptors on immune cells such as programmed cell death 1 and cytotoxic T-lymphocyte associated protein 4, down-regulates the T-cell-mediated immune response or immune checkpoints; antibodies that block these receptors tend to enhance antitumor immunity [11].

Such attempts as histopathologic typing of the tumors obscures the essential roles of such instability as well demonstrated by the onset and progression dynamics that affect both the tumor cells themselves and the tumor infiltrating DC.

It is beyond simple recognition of the neoplasm as an essentially progressive lesion that there evolves the dynamic systems of interactivities within proposed emergence of carcinogenesis as an established malignant tumor lesion.

The tumor microenvironment is important in cancer progression and immune checkpoint inhibitors are potential strategies in promoting the immune responses in cancer patients [12].

Tumor and DC interactivities thus can be recognized as paramount considerations within systems of ongoing carcinogenesis that progress as essentially unstable phenomena. Evidence has increasingly shown the potential of targeting neoantigens to generate effective clinical responses and in combination with checkpoint blockade monoclonal antibodies have demonstrated potent T-cell responses against these neoantigens [13]. It is this consideration that promotes and further enhances complexity of relative import in the ongoing process of permissiveness of the local microenvironment of the emerging tumor.

CONCLUSION

Consideration of the relative import of DC as beset by the emerging unstable carcinogenic tumor cell progenitors belies the evolutionary redefinition of a pathologic lesion that very early in tumorigenesis spreads to distant organs in the body.

The incorporation of tumor antigens is itself unstable and this has a profound import on the tumor-infiltrating DC. The added contexts of operability and inoperability of tumor neoantigens are further compounded by the emergence of instability as well demonstrated by systems of repeated redefinition of such tumor antigenicity on the one hand and of dendritic cell turnover that adds defining roles of DC cells in the context of cellular inactivity.

REFERENCES

[1] Peng M, Mo Y, Wang Y, Wu P, Zhang Y, Xiong F et al. "Neoantigen vaccine: an emerging tumor immunotherapy" *Mol Cancer* 2019;18(1):128.

[2] Wu X, Gu Z, Chen Y, Chen B, Chen W, Weng L et al. "Application of PD-1 blockade in cancer immunotherapy" *Comput Struct Biotechnol J* 2019;17:661-674.

[3] Ma Y, Shurin GV, Gutkin DW, Shurin MR "Tumor associated regulatory dendritic cells" *Semin Cancer Biol* 2012;22(4):298-306.

[4] Jakubowski CD, Azad NS "Immune checkpoint inhibitor therapy in biliary tract cancer (cholangiocarcinoma)" *Chin Clin Onco* 2020;9(1):2.

[5] Nosho K, Sukawa Y, Adachi Y, Ito M, Mitsubishi K, Kurihara H et al. "Association of Fusobacterium nucleatum with immunity and molecular alterations in colorectal cancer" *World J Gastroenterol* 2016;22(2):557-66.

[6] Orbegoso C, Murali K, Banerjee S "The current status of immunotherapy for cervical cancer" *Rep Pract Oncol Radiother* 2018;23(6):580-588.

[7] Saeed A, Park R, Al-Jumayli M, Al-Rajabi R, Sun W "Biologics, immunotherapy, and future directions in the treatment of advanced cholangiocarcinoma" *Clin Colorectal Cancer* 2019;18(2):81-90.

[8] Roberti MP, Yonekura S, Duong CPM, Picard M, Ferrere G, Tidjani Alou M et al. "Chemotherapy-induced ill crypt apoptosis and the ideal micro biome shape immunosurveillance and prognosis of proximal colon cancer" *Nat Med* 2020;26(6):919-931.

[9] Chen X, Pan X, Zhang W, Guo H, Cheng S, He Q et al. "Epigenetic strategies synergies with PD-L1/PD targeted cancer immunotherapies to enhance antitumor responses" *Acta Pharm Sin B* 2020;10(5):723-733.

[10] Yu Y, Zeng D, Ou Q, Liu S, Li A, Chen Y et al. "Association of survival and immune-related biomarkers with immunotherapy in patients with non-small cell lung cancer: a meta-analysis and

individual patient-level analysis" *JAMA Netw Open* 2019;2(7):e196879.

[11] Zhou G, Sprengers D, Boor PPC, Doukas M, Schutz H, Mancham S et al. "Antibodies against immune checkpoint molecules restore functions of tumor-infiltrating T cells in hepatocellular carcinomas" *Gastroenterology* 2017;153(4):1107-1119.

[12] Fathi M, Pustokhina I, Kuznetsov SV, Khayrullin M, Hojjat-Farsangi M, Karpisheh V et al. "T-cell immunoglobulin and ITIM domain, as a potential immune checkpoint target for immunotherapy of colorectal cancer" *IUBMB Life* 2021;73(5):726-738.

[13] Aldous AR, Dong JZ "Personalized neoantigeen vaccines: a new approach to cancer immunotherapy" *Bioorg Med Chem* 2018;26(10):2842-2849.

Chapter 10

SYSTEMS OF PREDETERMINATION OF CYTOKINE/CHEMOKINE ACTION TOWARDS CANCER ANTIGENICITY IN TERMS OF DENDRITIC CELL PLASTICITY

ABSTRACT

The promotional attributes of antigen processing are integral to a predetermined characterization of antigen presentation phenomena against cancer antigens as provided by dendritic cells. In such terms, redistribution of action of intracellular peptide molecules within dendritic cells attributes the overall recharacterization of systems of inducing predeterminants as provided by the ongoing continuum of DC subset processing of antigens. The functionality and dysfunctionality of DC mobility call into action the promotional induction of interdependence of cytokine action and chemokine determination as provided by systems of cooperative intercellularity.

Such a process is hence the attribute predetermination of plasticity phenomena of DC within contextual reference phenomena of interaction between intracellular and extracellular pathogens and of cancer antigens per se.

Introduction

The referral plasticity of dendritic cells (DC) is constantly evoked within the contextual maturational programs of these cells. DC sense the environment and process antigen for presentation as central to immune responses [1]. Within such microenvironments, DC evoke the evolving programs of maturation with regard in particular to peptide/MHC complexes and of a full panorama of costimulatory molecules. There is no consensus on how to manufacture DC vaccines [2]. In such terms, the complexity of the antigen presenting processes includes derivative dimensions of cooperative cross presentation to a cytotoxic cell series of components.

Evolutionary Context

The inclusive evolutionary pathways as depicted by response to both intracellular pathogens and to extracellular pathogenic stimuli allow for the exposure of peptide/MHC complexes situated on the cell surface membrane. Therapeutic targeting of DC continues to hold translational potential in combinatorial strategies [3]. Allogeneic-IgG-loaded and HLA-restricted neoantigen DC vaccines have robust anti-timor effects in mice [4].

In this regard, cytokines and also chemokines evoke induction phenomena as self-contained evolutionary patterns of cell damage and apoptotic cells, on the one hand, and to pathogenic molecular patterns in a series of inducing activation of T cells. Depletion of vancomycin-sensitive bacteria enhances the antitumor action of radiotherapy [5]. In such terms, production of induction programs in T cell activation is provoked as performance imaged dimensions as confirmed by distinct programs of maturation of the DC antigen-presenting roles.

Several approaches have been utilised for the evaluation for long-term anti-tumor immune responses by DC [6]. There appear to be opportunities for *in vitro* antigen loading of different DC subsets such as conventional DC and monocyte-derived DC [7].

Antigen Processing

The production for central roles of DC antigen-processing programs determines the whole evolutionary pathway progression as determined by a continuum process of maturation of the DC. In particular, the mannose receptor is a highly effective endocytic receptor involved in antigen delivery and possibly T cell differentiation and cellular activation [8]. It is further to such considerations that antigen processing is derived from the induction by cytokines in particular.

The processes of macropinocytosis, phagocytosis and receptor-dependent endocytosis are themselves a revealed complex of induced interactivity in terms that go beyond cell receptivity of antigen-specific T cell activation.

It is paramount consideration to view such complexity of activation pathways as terms of reference to ongoing interactive prominence of activation of T cells in particular. Plasmacytoid DC show an impaired response to Toll-like receptor 7/9 activation, decreased interferon alpha production and also contribute to an immunosuppressive tumor microenvironment [9]. Such promotional dimensions include the tolerogenic stimuli of T cells as dictated by antigen presentation of DC and as further generation of regulatory subsets of T lymphocytes.

Environment

Incremental evolutionary processes evolve within the inceptive environment of pathogenic molecules that are processed by DC. RNA vaccines constitute an attractive platform for cancer immunotherapy, with modifications to optimise mRNA vaccine stability and translational efficiency and for non-viral delivery [10].

It is further to such considerations that the fully detailed processes of antigen processing dominantly determine the contextual microenvironment of the subsequent phenomenon of antigen presentation by DC as professional and highly potent cells.

The incumbent character of DC is functionally susceptible to the emergence of partially mature antigen presenting cells within a continuum for further maturation pathway evolution. It is significant to view DC as prominent antigen-characterized programs that significantly redirect pathways of antigen presentation in terms of the powerful plasticity attributes of these cells. mRNA vaccines can be used to quickly target patient-specific neoantigens that are identified by analysing the tumor exome; *in vitro* manipulated cells can be transfected with mRNA encoding tumor associated antigens or else patient-derived T cells with mRNAs encoding chimeric antigen receptors that recognise directly a specific tumor antigen [11].

Plasticity of DC

Hence, plasticity is evoked as both phenotypic and functional profiles within the subsequent series of re-characterization of recognition programs of antigen. The performance determination of the environmental inflammatory milieu is significant in terms of the characterization of induced antigen processing as revealed by such attributes particularly of the stereotypic initiation of antigen processing that promotes in its turn the emergence of antigen presentation and repeated re-characterization.

Antigen Processing

DC are the most potent professional antigen-presenting cells and are unique to initiate, maintain and regulate the intensity of primary immune responses [12]. The fully evolved dimensions of such processing events are strict specific subset evolution of the DC as provided by systems of cross presentation and of selective activation of the CD4+ T lymphocytes.

The fusion of endosomes to the membranes of the endoplasmic reticulum in particular and the roles of the TAP1/2 transportation system of antigens are integral components within a complex intracellular microenvironment of cytosolic re-characterization. DC are well suited to activate T cells toward many types of antigens due to their potent costimulatory activity [13]. In such terms, the evolutionary attributes of intracellular transport and localization is paramount characterization of the antigen processing that dominantly determines attributes of the subsequent antigen presentation phenomenon.

PREDETERMINATION

Substantial predetermination of DC presentation of antigen is therefore a result of the inducing of the cell presentation in its own right.

It is significant to view dimensions of dynamic trafficking of the DC as terms of incremental dimensions as accumulative effects of cytokine action. The significant redistribution of effects of DC turnover as distributed within germinal centers and lymphoid follicles illustrates the performance induction as predetermined by the antigen processing machinery of the DC. It is significant in particular to elucidate such antigen processing as a prime functionality of the transporting systems within the cellular cytosol. It is further to such considerations that predetermination is an overall dominating series of influences that radically re-characterize the subsequent antigen presentation on a multi-repeated basis.

Future DC-based therapies involve genetic DC modification, the use of CD34+ precursors, direct tumor delivery of DC and the utilisation of tumor lysates or apoptotic cells to provide additional undefined antigens (14).

Conclusion

The overall dimensionality of systems of provoked induction of predetermined antigen processing by DC is hence a provoking term of reference within systems that proceed and further re-characterize both the innate and adaptive phases of the immune response. The performance attributes of such antigen processing are further illustrating as further predetermination of action of cytokines in particular. The chemokine influences are referral determinants of DC motility within systems for further inducing influences on DC. It is in terms of significant cellular interaction as provided in particular by gap junctions between cells that a proliferative response constitutes the basis for DC hyper-mobility as borne out by the inducing phenomena themselves. The character of such induction is provocative basis for predetermination of pathways of antigen processing within systems that come to activate T lymphocytes against cancer antigens.

References

[1] Kotsias F, Cebrian I, Alloatti A "Antigen processing and presentation" *Int Rev Cell Mol Biol* 2019;348:69-121.

[2] Sabado RL, Balan S, Bhardwaj N "Dendritic cell-based immunotherapy" *Cell Res* 2017;27(1):74-95.

[3] Gardner A, Ruffell B "Dendritic cells and cancer immunity" *Trends Immunol* 2016;37(12):855-865.

[4] Wang Y, Xiang Y, Xin VW, Wang XW, Peng XC, Liu XQ et al. "Dendritic cell biology and its role in tumor immunotherapy" *J Hematol Oncol* 2020;13(1):107.

[5] Uribe-Herranz M, Rafail S, Beghi S, Gil-de-Gomez L, Verginadis I, Bittinger K et al. "Gut microbiota modulate dendritic cell antigen presentation and radiotherapy-induced antitumor immune response" *J Clin Invest* 2020;130(1):466-479.

[6] Sadeghzadeh M, Bornehdeli S, Mohahammadrezakhani H, Abolghasemi M, Poursaei E, Asadi M, Zafari V et al. "Dendritic cell therapy in cancer treatment; the state-of-the-art" *Life Sci* 2020;254:117580.

[7] Huber A, Dammeijer F, Aerts JGJV, Vroman H "Current state of dendritic cell-based immunotherapy: opportunities for *in vitro* antigen loading of different DC subsets?" *Front Immunol* 2018;9:2804.

[8] Martinez-Pomares L "The mannose receptor" *J Leukoc Biol* 2012;92(6):1177-86.

[9] Mitchell D, Chintala S, Dey M "Plasmacytoid dendritic cell in immunity and cancer" *J Neuroimmunol* 2018;322:63-73.

[10] McNamara MA, Nair SK, Holl EK "RNA-based vaccines in cancer immunotherapy" *J Immune Res* 2015;2015:794528.

[11] Fiedler K, Lazzaro S, Lutz J, Rauch S, Heidenreich R "mRNA cancer vaccines" *Recent Results Cancer Res* 2016;209:61-85.

[12] Zhong H, Shurin MR, Han B "Optimizing dendritic cell-based immunotherapy for cancer" *Expert Rev Vaccines* 2007;6(3):333-45.

[13] Meidenbauer N, Andreessen R, Mackensen A "Dendritic cells for specific cancer immunotherapy" *Biol Chem* 2001;382(4):507-20.

[14] Esche C, Shurin MR, Lotze MT "The use of dendritic cells for cancer vaccination" *Curr Opin Mol There* 1999;1(1):72-81.

Chapter 11

EXOSOME SYSTEM PREFERENCES AS INTEGRAL TO THE IMMUNE RESPONSE AND IMMUNE NON-RESPONSE TO TUMOR NEOANTIGENS

ABSTRACT

System profiles are inherent dimensions of an integral immune responsiveness that includes the participation of cell injury in the origin and progression of carcinogenesis and tumor progression. The realization of injury to systems for impaired immune responses is a conceptual idealization of the roles of a homeostasis that is inherently aberrant. In such terms, ongoing systems for involvement of the immune response in tumor cell rejection are a potential distortion of increments of integral immune response and suppression. The derivation of dysfunctionality of tumor cell exosomal participation is an induction of the cell injury that gives rise to a series of neoantigens on the part of the tumor cells that spread primarily and only secondarily proliferate. The microenvironmental reconditioning is system characterization of such tumor spread potential that is realized as system preference dynamics.

Introduction

Exosomal production and series of functions include both immunostimulatory and immunosuppressive functionalities with a basic repertoire of induced secretion by both tumor cells and DC. Dendritic cell (DC)-derived exosomes are secreted by the sentinel antigen-presenting cells of the immune response; their composition includes surface expression of MHC-peptic complexes and costimulatory molecules and they facilitate immune cell-dependent tumor rejection [1]. In such terms, the ongoing basic cell biology of exosomal production and functionality/dysfunctionality include a realization of secretory activity that is integral also for the evolutionary utilization of antigen stimulation in cell-to-cell contact phenomena. Exosomes can impinge on signal transduction pathways and mediate signaling crosstalk, thus modulating cell-to-cell communication and macrophage activation and polarisation [2]. During antitumor immune response, DC-derived exosomes participate in antigen presentation [3].

In such terms, ongoing experiments on immune reactivity and non-reactivity seem to constitute a series of immunostimulatory roles that transgress the functional roles of T cells as borne out by systems of induced reproducibility.

Exosomes

The integral dimensions of exosomes as conveyors of antigens from tumor cells to DC is beset by the basic hierarchical confrontations of systems of inducible pathways as events culminating on both suppression and stimulation of a global immune response. Tumor exosome treatment suppresses the maturation and migration of DC and promotes immune suppression by DC [4]. In such terms, ongoing dimensions that constitute the nature of events inherent to exosome production and secretion would convey a realization of antigenic participation within systems for further involvement of an immune response to proliferating and spreading tumor cells. Exosomes are able to exert immunosuppression as well as trigger an anti-tumor response by presenting tumor antigens to DC [5].

CELL INJURY

The dimensionalization of injury to tumor cells may account for system preferences that incorporate the concrete confrontations of cell-to-cell contact. DC-derived exosomes constitute a new class of antitumor vaccines [6]. In such terms, the presence of FasL and TRAIL molecules on the membranes of exosomes would indicate a further system series within the exosomal repertoire as best evidenced by cross presentation of immune system roles.

The proportionalities of incongruent functionalities of exosomes are system profiles that participate within the proportional dimensions of exosomal membrane and proteolytic enzyme dysfunctions of these particles. A synapse is formed between interacting DC and vesicle transfer develops in the absence of free exosomes [7]. In terms that are ongoing participants of the induced immune response to tumor cells, the further participation of cellular injury is inherent dimension to the exosome that is integral to cytoskeletal dysfunctionality of both tumor cells and DC.

Exosome DNA is involved in priming tumor immunity and also regulates, in critical manner, check-point immunotherapy [8].

VARIABILITY OF CELL CONTACT

The incumbent involvement of exosomal inter-activities is complex variability of principal cell-to-cell contact within, however, a system profile of induced secretory activity as borne out by the enzymes and mediators contained within the exosomes. Immune cell-derived exosomes is capable of mediating crosstalk between innate and adaptive immunity and regulate cancer progression and spread; transfer of RNA, functional proteins, lipids and metabolites may take place *in vivo* [9].

The participation of injury to the profile dimensions of dysfunctional and functional attributes of exosomes encompasses the common phenomena of both DC and tumor cells towards the emergence of transfer dynamics of unresolved immune responses. Exosomes are derived from multi vesicular endosomes and can transfer membrane, cytosolic proteins, lipids and nucleotides and also micro RNAs [10].

It is the realization of cell injury as inherent to tumor cell biologic derivation constitutes the dimensions for further exosome production and function. It is within such terms of reference that the ongoing involvement of tumor cells not to induce immune responses that exosomes prove referable profiles for further tumor microenvironmental conditioning and reconditioning.

DEVELOPMENT

Incremental participation of the exosomal apparatus is hence a developmental aspect of the integral carcinogenesis phenomenon as carried forward by systems for impaired responses on the part of the immune system that is both stimulated and suppressed by cell-to-cell contact processes. The developmental increments of such injury are integral immune response to foreign antigen on the one hand and of system profiles for further participation in immune suppression. In such terms, ongoing evolutionary involvement is attribute setting within the immune systems of response or non-response.

The participation of cell injury in tumor cell biology is thus carried forward by the involvement of integral dynamics of inherent immune responses of a series of tumor-associated antigens. Exosomes derived from immature DC can modulate the immune response, but do not participate in direct T cell activation *in vitro* [11]. It is incumbent participation of cell biologic apparatus that defines the scope for the immune responses in the first instance. In such terms, ongoing dimensions for foreign-antigen recognition allow for a primarily permissive series of responses that include apoptosis of T lymphocytes in particular.

ANTIGENICITY

Dominating participants in inclusive dimensions of the immune response appear to be integral to the system profiles for transfer dynamics between systems for such recognition of antigenicity on the part of the immune system and of the DC. DC as immune cells are hence capable for the restoration of an immune milieu that is primarily plastic and undeniably not homeostatic.

In such terms, ongoing participation of injury to cells constitutes the potential for exosome formulation and secretion within systems of response and non-response on the part of the integral immune response. The mechanism and function of exosomes have transformed the understanding of cellular exchanges and the molecular events that underlie cancer progression [12].

SYSTEM PROFILES

The evidential participation of system profiles apply primarily to an immune system primarily constituted to suppress or activate recognition of foreign antigen. Antigen-specific CD8(+) T cells can regulate immune responses via T cell release of exosomes [13]. Exosomes from tumor cells may promote immunologic tolerance and even active immunosuppression [14]. In such terms, the ongoing involvement of system integration of immune responses is defining term in the confrontation of viable response or non-response of immune cells and of DC in particular.

Conclusion

System profile setting in the immune system is response to antigen within the integral conditioning of an immune suppression. In such terms, the potentiality for an immune-mediated rejection of tumor cells is beset by pathways for transfer as well illustrated by the reactivities arising from cell-to-cell contact with T lymphocytes. The incumbent transfer mechanics, as idealized by exosome production and functionality, include the suppressive elements of immune responses in general. In such terms, ongoing implications for an integral immune response include the evolutionary development of a microenvironmental milieu for the tumor within set limits for involvement of DC and T lymphocytes. The emergence of integers for an immune response include the emergence also of DC cells that maintain responsiveness of various immune cells in the face of carcinogenesis and tumor biology.

References

[1] Pitt JM, Andre F, Aigorena S, Soria J-C, Eggermont A, Kroemer G et al. "Dendritic cell-derived exosomes for cancer therapy" *J Clin Invest* 2016;126(4):1224-32.

[2] Baig MS, Roy A, Rajpoot S, Liu D, Savai R, Banerjee S et al. "Tumor-derived exosomes in the regulation of macrophage polarisation" *Inflamm Res* 2020;69(5):435-451.

[3] Wang Y, Xiang Y, Xin VW, Wang XW, Peng XC, Liu XQ et al. "Dendritic cell biology and its role in tumor immunotherapy" *J Hematol Oncol* 2020;13(1):107.

[4] Ning Y, Shen K, Wu Q, Sun X, Bai Y, Xie Y et al. "Tumor exosomes block dendritic cells maturation to decrease the T cell immune response" *Immunol Lett* 2018;199:36-43.

[5] Kahlert C, Kalluri R "Exosomes in tumor microenvironment influence cancer progression and metastasis" *J Mol Med* (Berl) 2013;91(4):431-7.

[6] Lu Z, Zuo B, Jing R, Gao X, Rao Q, Liu Z et al. "Dendritic cell-derived exosomes elicit tumor regression in autochthonous hepatocellular carcinoma mouse models" *J Hepatic* 2017;67(4):739-748.

[7] Rutland MK, Roberts EW, Cai E. Mujal AM, Marshuk K, Beppler C et al. "Visualizing synaptic transer of tumor antigens among dendritic cells" *Cancer Cell* 2020'37(6):786-799.

[8] Sharma A, Johnson A "Exosome DNA: critical regulator of tumor immunity and a diagnostic biomarker" *J Cell Physiol* 2020;235(3):1921-1932.

[9] Yan W, Jiang S "Immune cell-derived exosomes in the cancer-immunity cycle" *Trends Cancer* 2020;6(6):506-517.

[10] Seo N, Akiyoshi K, Shiku H "Exosome-mediated regulation of tumor immunology" *Cancer Sci* 2018;109(10):2998-3004.

[11] Quay BJC, O'Neill HC "The immunogenicity of dendritic cell-derived exosomes" *Blood Cells Mol Dis* 2005;35(2):94-110.

[12] Zhang L, Yu D "Exosomes in cancer development, metastasis, and immunity" *Biochim Biophs Acta Rev Cancer* 2019;1871(2):455-468.

[13] Xie Y, Zhang H, Li W, Deng Y, Munegowda MA, Chibbar R, Qureshi M et al. "Dendritic cells recruit T cell exosomes via exosomal LFA-1 leading to inhibition of CD8+ CTL responses through down regulation of peptide/MHC class I and Fas ligand-mediated cytotoxicity" *J Immune* 2010;185(9):5268-78.

[14] Wang K, Tang J "Tumor-derived exosomes and their roles in cancer" *Zhong Nan Da Xue Xao Yi Xue Ban* 2010;35(12):1288-92.

Chapter 12

CONSTITUTION OF A FAILED ANTITUMOR IMMUNE RESPONSE AS CARCINOGENESIS SUSTAINMENT

ABSTRACT

The constitutive provocations of an immature DC governing enhanced tumor cell proliferation and spread constitute effective further carcinogenesis as projected by systems of tumor cell derivation and progression. The developmental dynamics of an ineffective antitumor immune response constitute the elements for further progression of neoplastic growth that derives sustained stimulation in terms of the genesis of various tumor derived growth factors such as vascular endothelial growth factor. The involvement of vascular leukocytes is inciting element within the encompassed derivation of a lesion whose growth and spread is actively enhanced by the immature DC and as further proposed by systems of multilayers of DC dysfunctionality.

INTRODUCTION

The distinctive biologic traits of tumor-associated dendritic cells (DC) have indicated the potential perturbations of immature DC as these relate to a series of dysfunctional states in T-cell helper modulation against the tumor. M2 polarized tumor-associated macrophages and immature DC are centrally implicated in subversion of adaptive immunity and in inflammatory circuits that enhance tumor progression [1]. The various model systems indicate also the potential generation of regulatory T cells that tend to suppress antitumor activities by DC. Myeloid-derived suppressor cells are major inhibitors of immune effector cell function in tumors, and their differentiation is shaped by the tumor microenvironment [2]. The incremental dimensions of involved DC dysfunctional states relate to a multi-layered series of abnormalities in terms that further enhance tumor cell proliferation and spread. Chronic exposure of damage-associated molecular patterns, on the other hand, activates immature DC to transition to a mature phenotype [3].

Microenvironment

The particular enhancements of dysfunctional status of tumor microenvironmental DC indicate the relative contact dynamics of DC with naïve T cells in a manner that is incumbent to the further growth of the neoplasm. In such terms, immaturity of DC appears to suppress contact constitution in relative manner to T cells in the tumor microenvironment.

It is further to such considerations that the development of a failed immune response to tumor cell antigenicity is an acquired differential attribute that provokes further suppression of antitumor immune response. Immature myeloid cells induce immunosuppression through the expression of various cytokines, inhibition of lymphocyte homing, stimulation of other immunosuppressive cells, depletion of metabolites critical to T cell function, and expression of ectoenzymes regulating adenosine metabolism, and reactive species generation [4].

PERFORMANCE DYNAMICS

Performance dynamics are themselves incremental attributes that incriminate the disruption of differentiation processes of immature DC. It is further to such a phenomenon that potential incumbency of stimulation of T cytotoxic and helper cells varies with differential histomorphologic types of tumors, including for example ovarian epithelial tumors and breast ductal carcinomas.

It is the apparent distinctiveness of myeloid DC and of plasmacytoid DC differentiation processes that especially afflicts the dynamics of an antitumor immune response in a manner that particularly enhances suppressive regulatory T cell generation and activities. Tutors may impair antigen presentation, active negative costimulatory signals, and elaborate immunosuppressive factors [5].

In such manner, the conflicting contrasts of these two classes of DC modes of differentiation are hurdles in the generation and sustainment of an antitumor immune response.

It appears significant that the vascular endothelial cell growth factor in particular inhibits differentiation of DC to a fully mature immunotype and phenotype.

FAILED IMMUNE RESPONSE

In such manner, the ongoing genesis of a failed antitumor immune response arises as an expression of growth factors in general with the subsequent emergence of dysfunctional DC within expressly emerging tumor microenvironments. Dendritic cells otherwise play central roles in initiating, directing and regulating adaptive immune responses including tutor immunosurveillance [6].

The large populations of DC that can be generated from malignant ascitic fluids indicate the potential increments of DC within the encompassed derivative dimensions of tumors that additively enhance tumor growth rather than as a suppressing series of mechanisms against tumorigenesis. Also, immature dendritic cell/tumor cell fusions induce robust antitumor immunity [7].

In such terms, the increments in neoplastic growth are dependent and appear to sustain the maturity status of DC functionality and response to such neoplasms.

Increments of Tumor Growth and Spread

Tumor growth and angiogenesis depend on the presence of immature dendritic cells and hence promoted DC maturation may both augment the host immune response to the neoplasm and also suppress tumor angiogenesis [8], Provocative increments are hence a deliberately equated dimension with the biologic microenvironment of a neoplasm that suppresses effectively the antitumor immune response. In such terms, ongoing derivatives of differentiating tumor cells are themselves suppressive elements in the modulation of a failed antitumor immune response. The provocative stimulatory elements in the generation of regulatory T cells would encompass particular subsets of a highly heterogeneous DC series of multilayed dysfunctions as evidenced by microenvironmental classes of cells ranging from developmental to dysfunctional abnormalities.

In breast carcinoma, immature dendritic cells are found within the neoplasm, whereas mature dendritic cells are present peritumorally [9].

The dysfunctional axis of operative suppression of the antitumor immune response credits the ongoing process of such dysfunctionality of DC within the microenvironmental dynamics of a tumor that acquires, thus, the modulation of the immune system in terms of further carcinogenesis.

The potentiality of involvement of immature DC in carcinogenesis is beset by the tumor enhancing growth factors such as vascular endothelial growth factor in particular. In such terms, the ongoing neoplastic series of mechanisms arise in concert with the failed antitumor immune response in a manner that distinctively provokes the genesis of autonomous tumor cell proliferative bursts and spread of metastatic deposits within systemic organs.

Macrophages undergo a broad range of polarised activation states, and can both elicit tumor and tissue destruction and to promote tumor progression; they are also key elements in connecting cancer with inflammation [10].

M2 polarisation of murine peritoneal macrophages stimulates regulatory cytokine production and inhibits T-cell proliferation [11].

Such a paradoxical series of events in neoplastic cell proliferation and spread are descriptive models of operability that subsist to the generation of a failed antitumor immune response that arises in active participation to various models of tumor cell proliferation and spread. In such terms, the ongoing dynamics of incumbency are relative proportions to the emergence of carcinogenesis as primal derivative of the immaturity of the DC in the tumor microenvironment.

Dysfunctionality and Immaturity of Dendritic Cells

It is significant to view the genesis of a failed antitumor immune response as symptomatic of a series of dysfunctionalities that express directly and in multilayered manner the dysfunctionalities of DC as emerging and reemerging cellular immaturity.

Conclusion

Dysfunctional and immature DC are harbingers of a failed antitumor immune response as descriptively outlined by various conceptual models of failed antitumor immune responses. The dynamics of DC immaturity are both generative and consequent motives within a tumor microenvironment that is beset by a tumor lesion that grows, proliferates and spreads as dynamics of regulatory T cell activity. In such terms, ongoing dysfunctionalities of DC immaturity come to constitute carcinogenesis events in their own right and within the abbreviated dimensions of ongoing processes of various failed contact dimensions with helper and cytotoxic T cells.

In a manner of constitutive reappraisal, the dimensions of modulation of a failed antitumor immune response constitute the realization of enhanced tumor growth and spread.

REFERENCES

[1] Mantovani A, Sozzani S, Locati M, Allavena P, Sica A "Macrophage polarisation: tumor-associated macrophages as a paradigm for polarized M2 mononuclear phagocytes" *Trends Immunol* 2002;23(11):549-55.

[2] Tcyganov E, Mastio J, Chen E, Gabrilovich DI "Plasticity of myeloid-derived suppressor cells in cancer" *Curr Opin Immunol* 2018;51:76-82.

[3] Zhou J, Wang G, Chen Y, Wang H, Hua Y, Cai Z "Immunogenic cell death in cancer therapy: present and emerging inducers" *J Cell Mol Med* 2019;23(8):4854-4865.

[4] Groth C, Hu X, Weber R, Fleming V, Altevogt P, Utikal J et al. "Immunosuppression mediated by myeloid-derived suppressor cells (MDSCs) during tumour progression" *Br J Cancer* 2019;120(1):16-25. 148

[5] Rabinovich GA, Gabrilovich D, Sotomayor EM "Immunosuppressive strategies that are mediated by tumor cells" *Annu Rev Immune* 2007;25:267-96.

[6] Strioga M, Schijns V, Powell DJ Jr, Pasukoniene V, Dobrovolskiene N, Michalek J "Dendritic cells and their role in tumor immunosurveillance" *Innate Immune* 2013;19(1):98-111.

[7] Takeda A, Homma S, Okamoto T, Kufe D, Ohno T "Immature dendritic cell/tumor cell fusions induce potent antitumor immunity" *Eur J Clin Invest* 2003;33(10):897-904.

[8] Fainaru O, Almog N, Yung CW, Nakai K, Montoya-Zavala M, Abdullahi A et al. "Tumor growth and angiogenesis are dependent on the presence of immature dendritic cells" *FASEB J* 2010;24(5):1411-8.

[9] Bell D, Chomarat P, Broyles D, Netto G, Harb GM, Lebecque S et al. "In breast carcinoma tissue, immature dendritic cells reside within the tumor, whereas mature dendritic cells are located in peritumoral areas" *J Exp Med* 1999:190(10):1417-26. 149.

[10] Mantovani A, Sica A, Allavena P, Garlanda C, Locati M "Tumor-associated macrophages and the related myeloid-derived suppressor cells as a paradigm of the diversity of macrophage activation" *Hum Immunol* 2009;70(5):325-30.

[11] Oishi S, Takano R, Tamura S, Tani S, Iwaizumi M, Hamaya Y et al. "M2 polarization of murine peritoneal macrophages induces regulatory cytokine production and suppresses T-cell proliferation" *Immunology* 2016;149(3):320-328.

Chapter 13

MULTIPLE MODELS OF FAILED IMMUNE RESPONSES REDEFINE CARCINOGENESIS

ABSTRACT

Dimensionality is the true nature of the multiple models of representation of a failed immune response to the tumor. In such terms, the derivative dimensions of neoantigenicity are remarkable constitution of integral pools of emerging tumor cells that evade the immune response in terms inherently reflecting the process of carcinogenesis. In such terms, the equivocal dimensions for further reconstitution reflect the dominant nature of the failure mechanisms of the antitumor immune response, as well exemplified by growth factor actions and of apoptosis of dendritic cells.

INTRODUCTION

The descriptive reports of evasive behavior from immune surveillance as defined by tumor cell behavior constitute the intermediary constitution of realization of suppressive dendritic cell (DC) action in modes of impaired DC maturation and of active DC apoptosis.

Lack of CD103+ DC within the tumor microenvironment resists the effector antitumor T cell response, promoting immune escape [1]. In such terms, ongoing constitution of realization of anergy and of immune tolerance indicate the modulatory action of, primarily, system pathways of suppression drawn by the escape mechanisms of interacting innate and adaptive immune systems. Immunogenic cell death appears to constitute a prominent pathway for activation of antitumor immune systems [2]. The successful development of effective innate immune activators would expand the fraction of patients responding to immunotherapy, as with checkpoint blockade antibodies [3].

In a further realization of systemic suppression of DC, there evolves the escape systems of apoptosis within systems of progressive adaptation that primarily target impaired generation of progenitor cells derived from hematopoietic tissues and of secondary lymphoid organs.

Recombination

In such terms, the descriptive recombinatorial systems of apoptotic DC death is an appropriate pathway expression as derived from various modulating factors as well depicted by the action of various cytokines and growth factors secreted not only by tumor cells but also especially by DC. During the process of cross-presentation tumor derived antigens are presented to CD8+ T cells by Batf3-dependent CD8a+/XCR1+ classical dendritic cells [4]. In the involvement of such complexity there arises the emergence of immature generation of DC dysfunction by circulating peripheral blood monocytes in constitutive expression of a failed antitumor immune response. Immune checkpoint blockade serves to reverse T cell exhaustion but DC are still required to prime, activate and direct the T cells in targeting tumor cells [5].

MONOCYTES

The system profile modulations of monocytic cell action are hence simple and relatively effective pathways; these constitutionally evoke the incremental dimensions of tolerance of immune cells that further promote suppression in the generation of DC as expressive induction especially of apoptosis within the additional domains of anergic tolerance to tumor cell antigenicity. There is an urgent need for biomarkers to choose the optimal candidates for immunotherapy in terms of efficacy and tolerance [6].

In such terms, ongoing systems of profile redefinition of the antitumor immune response are pathways of cell suppression of immune response that radically constitute the various intermediate reconstitution of such immune response in various highly effective pathways of immune suppression. Attempts are being made to target the Stimulator of Interferon Genes (STING) as immunotherapy of cancer by modulating the tumor microenvironment and induce type 2 interferon production [7].

GROWTH FACTORS

The incremental growth of immune responsiveness has been equivocally equated with a decreased effectiveness of DC as participants against growth factor functionality and dysfunctionality. In cross-priming, where DC activate CD8+ T cells by presenting exogenous antigens onto Major Histocompatibility Complex class I, CD8+ T cell immunity as well as tolerance are actively induced [8]. In such terms, the measure of incumbent nonresolution of system pathways of an effective antitumor immune response constitutes the failed redefinition of interactions between the innate and adaptive pathways of immune surveillance. The added system reconstitutions of various intermediate mediators are well defined by exemplary action of various tumor derived growth factors such as vascular endothelial growth factor in the first instance.

Such a scenario is well exemplified as system reproduction that is unfaithful in terms of constitutive representation. As such there emerge a series of modeled pathways that decry the terms of remodulation in terms beyond simple antigenic stimulation of both innate and adaptive immune systems. Antitumor immunity directed by intratumor DC contributes to efficacy of anthracycline-based chemotherapy against tumors [9].

Reconstitution

Reconstitution efforts on the part of the immune response to tumors is a centrally operative system to the redefinition of the antitumor immune status in a given cancer patient. Defined innate immune interactions in cancer include recognition by NK cells, NKT cells and gamma-delta T cells and also by dendritic cells and macrophages reacting to damage-associated molecular patterns [10]. Such terms of reference constitute an attempted rehabilitation of such immune responses within the constitutional reappraisal of an immune system that maladapts to the ongoing shedding of tumor cells in the local microenvironment and into the lymphatic and systemic circulations.

A reappraisal phenomenon of the failed antitumor immune response is hence a description depiction of an immune response beyond simple appraisal systems of continuous exposure of tumor antigens that however operates within suppressed immune surveillance.

Multiple Model Generation

Multi-models of attempted reconstitution of a failed immune response are a centrally operative mechanism in the redefinition of pathway recognition. The detection of danger signals, including DNA and RNA, by DC in cancers is essential for eliciting host defence but the molecular sensors for recognising danger signals and for eliciting anticancer immune responses remain unclear [11]. In terms beyond antigenicity, apoptosis of mature DC cells is both suppressive and also attempted reconstitution of the antitumor immune response. Multiple templates for such potential reconstitution of the immune surveillance are recognizable within terms for further remodeling of the immune response as constituted by the action of various cytokines, growth factors and gangliosides.

The soluble and cell surface molecules expressed by various tumor cells and host cells represent a potential stimulus for the ongoing remodeled pathways towards a new or novel interpretation of the tissue injury prerogative. The system representation of tissue and cell injury stimulates an attempted antitumor immune response that derives its effective reconstitution within terms of relative reference to a proliferating pool of tumor cells that primarily spreads as invoked by constitutive pathways of response on the one hand and of nonresponse to tumor cell antigenicity. The host STING pathway operates at the interface of cancer and immunity and senses cytosolic tumor derived DNA within tumor-infiltrating DC [12].

NEOANTIGENS

Models of immune response are hence responses to neoantigens as provoked by a variable increment in tumor cell pools that derive their dysfunctionality primarily in terms of the failure of the antitumor immune response.

The incremental activities of tumor cell pools incriminate the models of attempted reconstitution that encompass the nature of the initial carcinogenesis as carried forward by such failed antitumor immune response in the first instance. Engineering monocyte-derived DC to produce interferon-alpha enhances promotion of adaptive and innate anti-timor immune effector functions [13]. It is within the system profiles of multiple models of immune reconstitution that there emerges a representation of failed elimination of tumor cell pools that invoke further modeling attempts of immune response.

The loss of faithful representation of tumor cell antigenicity hence emerges within systems of representation of multiple models of the immune response. Within the plethora of cytokines and growth factors there emerge multi-dimensional mediators ranging from costimulatory molecules, suppressors and inducers within pathway representation and reconstitution. In such terms, the incremental dimensions for attempts at immune response are inhibitory moments for a fidelity that is both suppressive and potentially stimulatory.

Conclusion

Stimulation and suppression of the antitumor immune response are indicative of multiple profiles for attempted reconstitution. Tumor antigenicity is not a purely cellular phenomenon but the constitutive integration of entire tumor cell pools within systems of presentation and representation. In such terms, multiple models of reconstitution are attempts of reinterpretation of pathway progression as projected by the carcinogenesis that provokes further neoantigenicity. The incremental dimensions are projected by tumor cell spread systemically rather than by the high proliferative activities of the emerging tumor cell pools that constitute the profile reconstitution of a lesion that incrementally establishes a failed antitumor immune response.

References

[1] Spranger S, Dai D, Horton B, Gajewski TF "Tumor-residing Batf3 dendritic cells are required for effector T cell trafficking and adoptive T cell therapy" *Cancer Cell* 2017;31(5):711-723.

[2] Kroemer G, Galluzzi L, Kepp O, Zitvogel L "Immunogenic cell death in cancer therapy" *Annu Rev Immunol* 2013;31:51-72.

[3] Corrales L, Matson V, Flood B, Spranger S, Gajewski TF "Innate immune signaling and regulation in cancer immunotherapy" *Cell Res* 2017;27(1):96-108.

[4] Theisen DJ, Davidson JT 4th, Briseno CG, Gargaro M, Lauron EJ, Wang Q et al. "WDFY4 is required for cross-presentation in response to viral and tumor antigens" *Science* 2018;362(6415):694-699.

[5] Saxena M, Bhardwaj N "Re-emergence of dendritic cell vaccines for cancer treatment" *Trends Cancer* 2018;4(2):119-137.

[6] de Gooijer CJ, Borm FJ, Scherpereel A, Baas P "Immunotherapy in malignant pleural mesothelioma" *Front Oncol* 2020;10:187.

[7] Corrales L, Gajewski TF "Molecular pathways: targeting the stimulator of interferon genes (STING) in the immunotherapy of cancer" coin. *Cancer Res* 2015;21(21):4774-9. 161

[8] Fu C, Zhou L, Mi QS, Jiang A "DC-based vaccines for cancer immunotherapy" *Vaccines* (Basel) 2020;26;8(4):706.

[9] Vacchelli E, Ma Y, Baracco EE, Sistigu A, Enot DP, Pietrocola F et al. "Chemotherapy-induced antitumor immunity requires formyl peptide receptor 1" *Science* 2015;350(6263):972-8.

[10] Woo SR, Corrales L, Gajewski TF "Innate immune recognition of cancer" *Annu Rev Immunol* 2015;33:445-74.

[11] Rivera Vargas T, Benoit-Lizon I, Apetoh L "Rationale for stimulator of interferon genes-targeted cancer immunotherapy" *Eur J Cancer* 2017;75:86-97.

[12] Corrales L, McWhirter SM, Dubinsky TW Jr, Gajewski TF "The host STING pathway at the interface of cancer and immunity" *J Clin Invest* 2016;126(7):2404-11.

[13] Willemen Y, Van den Bergh JM, Lion E, Anguille S, Roelandts VA, Van Acker HH et al. "Engineering monocyte-derived dendritic cells to secrete interferon-alpha enhances their ability to promote adaptive and innate anti-tumor immune effector functions" *Cancer Immunol Immunother.* 2015;64(7):831-42.

Chapter 14

EFFECT DOMINANCE OF INTEGRAL CYTOKINE/CHEMOKINE NETWORKS IN TUMOR CELL ANTIGENICITY RESPONSE

ABSTRACT

The identity character and nature of whole integral networks of cytokines and chemokines are core mechanistic profiles within the phenomenal evolution of tumor cell antigenicity. The mechanistic attributes of such networks operate in specifically directed pathways of cooperative dimensions, as carried forward by systems of tumor cell and Dendritic Cell (DC) antigen presentation. In such terms, ongoing involvement in evolution of tumor cell antigenicity is integrative participation within the migratory and priming attributes of DC as carried forward by systems of DC antigen loading and presentation. The integral nature of cytokine/chemokine networks is primarily localised within the tumor microenvironment, but also as multi-system identity processes of antigen-recognition patterns, as conveyed by DC antigen loading and by T lymphocyte priming.

INTRODUCTION

The manipulation of tumor antigens and of tumor cell lysates, together with transfection techniques, utilising whole tumor cell genomes or mRNA, illustrate the huge potential for development of activated cytotoxic T lymphocytes in generating dendritic cell-based vaccines against a variety of cancers. The incumbent involvement of DC vaccines is derived inference in the quest for specific antitumor immune responses that operate within the sphere of subsequent potential necrosis of tumor cells, including metastatic and advanced cancer lesions. In such terms, the ex vivo generation of tumor antigen-loaded DC is particularly effective in inducing an antitumor immune response, without, however, eliciting objective tumor regression, in the majority of treated patients.

Myeloid -derived suppressor cells are major regulators of antitumor immune response [1]. The determined main factors involved in the lack of preexisting tumor T cell infiltration is essential for the utilisation of adapted algorithms of treatment for cold tumors [2].

The dimensions of cooperative HLA-restricted tumor antigen presentation, and the emergence of multi-pathway induction of an antitumor immune response, thus necessitate co-accessory stimulatory molecules and an essential cytokine milieu, within the tumor microenvironment, as postulated by seemingly diverse components of the naive T lymphocyte repertoire. B7-H1, a costimulatory molecule, is implicated in regulating cellular and humeral immune responses through the PD-1 receptor on activated T and B lymphocytes [3].

It is significant to view the ongoing pathways that crosstalk with the dynamics of generation of mature, actively functional DC, as indeed projected by the phenomena observed in the ex vivo generation of these antigen-presenting cells. In such terms, the ongoing privileged component pathways converge on naive T lymphocytes in the context of a realised series of dimensions that should target the tumor cells. Immunologic memory is defined quantitative and qualitative enhancement of immune response upon rechallenge;

Natural killer cells are able to remember inflammatory cytokine milieus that imprint persistent non-antigen-specific effector function [4]. In such manner, the availability of a series of cytokines, in particular Interleukin-12p70, in a manner that would transform such dynamics, is borne out by objective immune responsiveness. Chimeric antigen receptor T cells have been utilised to overcome tumor microenvironmental immune suppression involving such mechanisms as poor locating ability, immunosuppressive cells, chemokines, cytokines, immunosuppressive checkpoints, metabolic factors, loss of tumor antigen, and antigen heterogeneity [5].

SPECIFICITY

The specificity for an immune response to various tumor antigens includes the susceptibility dimensions as presented by the tumor cells, and the ongoing processes of tumor cell proliferation, in the *in vivo* dimensions of distribution of the DC within the tumor microenvironment.

In such terms, the ongoing process of sensitisation of the DC, as projected by systems of contrasting immature and mature DC and of the Regulatory T cells, also incorporates an essential series of roles for cytokines and of the chemokine receptor CCR7, and the Toll-like receptors in general. It is significant to view the system network participation of the integral immune system within encompassed dynamics of cooperative co-stimulatory molecules, and of pattern molecular recognition pathways, as these further substantiate the dynamics of migratory DC to the paracortex of the draining lymph nodes. Bispecific T-cell engagers enhance the immune response to neoplasms by retargeting T cells to tumor cells [6].

PATHWAY NON-RESOLUTION

Pathway non-resolution in the elicitation of such immune responses to tumor antigens, is a core concept in the observed turnover of DC pathways, especially in terms of anergy and of tolerance phenomena. The derivative dimensions of such non-resolution of targeting events to tumor antigen, is a significant and overwhelming pathway derivative as borne out by the proliferating neoplastic cells.

In such terms, the ongoing participation of contrasting dynamics is an essential outcome determinant within systems of turnover and also of migration of the DC. The effector arm of the immune system induces both antigen-specific Th cells and cytotoxic T cells, the generation of long lasting immunity, and a Th1 phenotype resulting in epitope spreading; Th1 cells activate antigen-presenting cells and induce production of antibodies that can enhance the uptake of tutor cells into DC [7].

It is further to such considerations that the presence of targeting modules by DC, that potentially converge on tumor cells, is akin to the core phenomenon of DC targeting of naive T lymphocyte subsets, particularly with regard to the cytotoxic T lymphocytes.

The derivative pathways of ongoing processing of tumor antigen are initiated by the highly phagocytic immature DC that, subsequently, mature to potent antigen-presenting cells. The T lymphocytes are themselves highly dynamic, and these coordinate in terms of specific response to antigen-presenting tumor cells.

Generation of specific tumor antigens correlates with a DC series of cell subtypes within the ongoing cytokine milieu, that itself evolves in its own right.

Cytokines modulate the genesis of new neoplasms and is mediated by regulating antigen-specific antitumor responses and activation of inflammation and innate resistance; a great effort has been carried out to exploit this antitumor potential [8]. In such terms, the variety of antigen presentation mechanisms is integral to a network series of construction phenomena, that participate within systems of antigen recognition and of anti-antigen immune response. A vaccine prepared by transfer of DNA from the neoplasm into a highly immunogenic cell line can encompass the array of tumor antigens that characterise that particular lesion [9]. It is significant to view the dimensions, for further growth of the cancer lesion, as derived participation of a series of cytokines that promote DC maturation without, however, provoking a non-responsive terminal differentiation state of the DC.

The particular attributes of system networks are reflective influence in the creation of dynamics of both antigen presentation and of stimulation of naive T lymphocytes.

The tumor microenvironment can prevent expansion of tumor antigen-specific helper and cytotoxic T cells, and instead enhance production of pro-inflammatory cytokines, and growth factors, with the generation of suppressive cell populations [10]. In such terms, the ongoing involvement of tumor antigenicity is inclusive formula in the generation of cytokine responsiveness and of their converging targeting of the proliferating tumor cells.

CONCLUSION

The whole series of hurdles in effective induced tumor cell regression is an abnormal participation of actively migratory DC subsets that are integrated within constitutive networks for cytokine action. The pliable interplay between immune and malignant cells is organised in phases of elimination, equilibrium and escape of the tumor cells [11]. The derivative elements of participation are compound influence in that the targeting stimulation of secretion of specific cytokines and of chemokines is core phenomenon in the evolution of the tumor cell antigenicity. The DC involvement, as professional antigen-presenting cells, is itself integral to such large scale networks of cytokine and chemokine action.

The realisation of effective antitumor response is, hence, inherent to the operative cytokine dimensions of response and action, within the tumor microenvironment.

The discernment for the overall immune response is, hence, derivative phenomenon that arises as cytokine attributes in the generation, also, of the antigen-loaded DC in the first instance. Tumor evasion of antigen detection by cell-surface receptors is one of the hallmarks of cancer [12]. In such terms, the further promotion of cytokine milieu is core phenomenon in the recognition of tumor cell antigenicity. The compound dimensions for further involvement of antigenic profiles contribute to patterns of molecular recognition that arise beyond the context of initial DC antigen presentation. The derivative priming of naive T lymphocytes is, itself, derived from cytokine network mechanisms of induction and participation in such tumor cell antigenicity.

REFERENCES

[1] Bronte V, Brandau S, Chen SH, Colombo MP, Frey AB, Greten TF et al. "Recommendations for myeloid-derived suppressor cell nomenclature and characterisation standards" *Nat Commun* 2016;7:12150.

[2] Bonaventura P, Shekarian T, Alcazer V, Valladeau-Guilemond J, Valsesia-Wittman S, Amigorena S et al. "Cold tumors: a therapeutic challenge for immunotherapy" *Front Immunol* 2019;10:168.

[3] Dong H, Strome SE, Salomao DR, Tamura H, Hirano F, Flies DB et al. "Tumor-associated B7-H1 promotes T-cell apoptosis: a potential mechanism of immune evasion" *Nat Med* 2002;8(8):793-800.

[4] Cerwenka A, Lanier LL "Natural killer cell memory in infection, inflammation and cancer" *Nat Rev Immunol* 2016;16(2):112-23.

[5] Zhao Z, Xiao X, Saw PE, Wu W, Huang H, Chen J et al. "Chimeric antigen receptor T cells in solid tumors: a war against the tumor microenvironment" *Sci China Life Sci* 2020;63(2):180-205.

[6] Huehis AM, Coupet TA, Sentman CL "Bispecific T-cell engagers for cancer immunotherapy" *Immunol Cell Biol* 2015;93(3):390-6.

[7] Kutson KL, Disis ML "Tumor antigen-specific T helper cells in cancer immunity and immunotherapy" *Cancer Immunol Immunother* 2005;54(8):721-8.

[8] Salazar-Onfray F, Lopez MN, Mendoza-Naranjo A "Paradoxical effects of cytokines in tumor immune surveillance and tumor immune escape" *Cytokine Growth Factor Rev* 2007;18(1-2)"171-82.

[9] Lichtor T, Glick RP "Immunogene therapy" *Adv Exp Med Biol* 2012;746:151-65.

[10] Finn OJ "Immuno-oncology: understanding the function and dysfunction of the immune system in cancer" *Ann Oncol* 2012;23 Suppl 8 (suppl 8):viii6-9.

[11] Cali B, Molon B, Viola A "Tuning cancer fate: the unremitting role of host immunity" *Open Biol* 2917; 7(4):170006.

[12] Guillerey C, Huntington ND, Smyth MJ "Targeting natural killer cells in cancer immunotherapy" *Nat Immunol* 2016;17 (9):1025-36.

Chapter 15

Incongruent Dislocation of Epitope Spread as Immunosuppression Dynamics of Tumor Cell Clones

Abstract

System profile indices of presenting dynamics of antigenicity implicate the turnover of neoplastic cells in terms of the incongruent dislocation of epitope spread of the neoantigens as dictated by clonality and by subsequent reconstitution of the lesion subpopulations through proliferation. The evolutionary profiles that are projected to the responding pathway recognition are integral to systems of emergence of the epitope participation as strict incongruence of performance dynamics of epitope spread within the tumor lesions. It is such turnover of whole clones of tumor cells that allows for emergence of incongruent epitope spread and as dictated by a mounting immune response.

The incremental dimensions for further tumor cell proliferation is hence a derived biologic attribute of the clonal dimensions for further incongruent epitope spread. The performance dynamics of the anti-tumor immune response are hence derivative of incongruent dislocation of antigen presentation, on the one hand, and of dynamics of clonality biology of the tumor lesion. It is further to such considerations that ongoing attempts at reconstitution of the immunogenic profile of the tumor cell clones implicate integral suppressive attributes of the tumor microenvironment as projected by abnormal dynamics of emergence of Dendritic Cell-derived antigen presentation.

Introduction

The interplay of genetically modified dendritic cells (DC) with immunostimulatory molecules and cytokines involves a reappraisal dimension within systems of immune response to cancer cells. In such measure, the provoked dimensions of system pathways that are involved include the stimulation of the DC as further pathway effectiveness, as borne out by the mounting immune response in absence of clinical anti-tumor response.

Inflammation-induced suppression of cytotoxic CD8+ T-lymphocytes activate a tumor-enhancing mechanisms [1]. In such terms, the ongoing involvement of the stimulated immune response to cancer cell epitopes implicates the realization of multi-faceted response on the part of the immune system, that can follow amplified production of antigen as presented to DC.

Blocking of the Transforming Growth Factor-beta along with immune checkpoint therapy increases T-helper1 subsets and enhances expansion of CD8+ T cells that improves survival [2].

Pathway Modulation

Involvement of the dimensionalized pathway modulations of the immune response re-characterize the cancer cell immune response as borne out by the evolutionary modification of genetic modification of DC. Large numbers of tissue-resident memory cells are related to better clinical outcomes in cancer patients [3].

Pathway incongruity is further accentuated by the development of gene transfection and by the mRNA transfection of DC.

Incremental augmentation of IL-12 and IL-18 production is counter-balanced by suppression of tumor-secreted soluble factors within the tumor and especially within the tumor microenvironment. Layilin, a C-type lectin domain-containing membrane glycoprotein, integrates with a molecular pathway in exhausted or dysfunctional CD8+ T-cells that enhances cellular adhesiveness to maintain their anti-tumor cytotoxicity [4]. Such dimensions incur the evolutionary and alternate pathways as directly modulated by DC maturation and antigen presentation. Tumor heterogeneity and clonal cooperation affect the immune selection of Interferon-gamma-signaling mutant tumor cells and contribute to immunotherapy resistance [5]. Free major histocompatibility complex presentation is further amplified as directed by induction pathways of the anti-cancer immune responses. Such immunity to tumor cell epitopes involves the realization of dimensionalized pathways that fail as clinical responsiveness.

The incumbent emergence phenomena of clinical non-responsiveness allows for the failed clinical regression of the tumor cells that are immunosuppressed, and as further attested to by the systems of non-emergence arrays of participating immune/tumor cell interactions.

ARRAYS OF IMMUNE RESPONSIVENESS

The participation of whole arrays of potential immune response accounts for the clinical failure in response to single molecular types of induction of the DC. Dual blockade of CD47 and HER2 eliminate radio resistant breast carcinoma cells through anti-phagocytosis conjugated with HER2-induced proliferation [6]. In such measure, the further promotional implications allow for regulatory T cells to suppress the immunogenicity of tumor cell populations that involve the overall emergence of the epitope exposure. The development of participation of immunostimulatory molecules and of cytotoxic T cells and cytokines, in a manner of emergence of subsequent clinical response, bespeak for the critical need to re-characterize in detail the generic modulatory roles in immune response.

FACS single cell index sorting is highly reliable and determines immune phenotypes of clonally proliferating T cells [7]. System pathway dimensions are critical evolutionary series of arrays as provided by the emergence dynamics of epitope exposure and spread.

The pathway recognition constitutes the core phenomenon of dynamic emergence profiles for DC participation in the anti-cancer response.

The strict definition of system profiles include the dimensional recognition of tumor antigens as provided by subsequent evolution of epitope definition. It is clearly the incongruent emergence of epitope recognition and of failed immuno-stimulation that accounts for the failure of clinical tumor regression in the face of a mounting anti-tumor immune response. In such terms, emergence of epitope presentation by DC is paramount consideration as profiles projected by induction pathways that progress in the face of epitope spread. The incongruence in participation of immunogenicity allows for the emergence of epitopes, as dictated by a poor anti-tumor response, clinically and pathologically.

Sensitization to immune checkpoint blockade occurs through activation of a STAT1/NK axis in the tumor microenvironment and provides a biomarker-driven approach to patient monitoring to determine whether benefit from treatment is possible [8].

CONGRUENCE DISLOCATION

The congruency-dislocated correlates of failed anti-tumor regression response redefine the dynamics of emergent immune response. In such terms, the repeated multi-faceted epitope emergence as presenting molecules inherent to the anti-tumor immune response allows for the participation of epitope spread per se as further modifications of the tumor cell pathogenesis.

In further consideration of incongruent epitope spread, dynamics of emergent pathway reconstitution allow for permissiveness as dictated by the overall integrity of the immune response. The development of emergence of antigen presentation is hence a basic biologic attribute of the epitope spread phenomenon. Such considerations are dynamic reconstitution of immunogenicity as dictated by the overall emergence of spread of epitopes as pronounced by the tumor cell biology of immune evasion.

The genesis for the simple antigenicity profiles for participation in anti-tumor immune response fails in terms of such emergence as direct correlates of the dynamics of the initial carcinogenesis pathways in tumor cell generation. Furthermore, the identity characteristics for involvement of effaced antigenicity of whole groups of tumor cells is incumbent to the evolutionary spread of epitopes, as further refined by systems of antigen recognition by the integral immune response.

Cancer regression and autoimmunity occur in patients subsequent to clonal repopulation with anti-tumor lymphocytes [9]. It is crucial to consider a neoplasm not simply as a clone of malignant cells but as a complex structure with multidirectional flow of information between the tumor cells and the multiple other cell types and extracellular matrix participants [10].

CONCLUSION

Performance dynamics are profile projections for a mounting immune response in the face of failed clinical tumor regression.

In such terms, strict considerations of emergence of epitope recognition and presentation belie the evolutionary dynamics of epitope spread as dictated by systems of progression as emergent clones of antigen presentation by both tumor cells and of DC. The realization of dynamics of turnover of whole clones of variant antigenicity of the tumor cells is further constitution of clonal biology as projected by neoplastic lesions. The pronounced biology of tumor cell turnover is dictated participant within systems of immunogenicity by various subtypes of DC, on the one hand, and of presentation dynamics of epitope spread. In such terms, the realization of a mounting immune response correlates with an incongruent response on the part of tumor cells that proliferate in strict terms of clonal expansion of the system profiles for further tumor cell proliferation. Within such biologic context, the emergence of neo-antigenicity is integral to the dynamics of the initial carcinogenesis that establishes the antigen presentation by the DC.

References

[1] Shalapour S, Lin XJ, Bastian IN, Brain J, Burt AD, Aksenov AA et al. "Inflammation-induced IgA+ cells dismantle anti-liver cancer immunity" *Nature* 2017;551(7680):340-345.

[2] Jiao S, Subudhi SK, Aparicio A, Ge Z, Guan B, Miura Y et al. "Differences in tumor microenvironment dictate T helper lineage polarization and response to immune checkpoint therapy" *Cell* 2019;179(5):1177-1190.

[3] Clarke J, Panwar B, Madrigal A, Singh D, Gujar R, Wood O et al. "Single-cell transcriptomic analysis of tissue-resident memory T cells in human lung cancer" *J Exp Med* 2019;216(9):2128-2149.

[4] Mahuron KM, Moreau JM, Glasgow JE, Boda DP, Pauli ML, Gouirand V et al. "Layilin augments integrin activation to promote antitumor immunity" *J Exp Med* 2020;217(9):e20192080.

[5] Williams JB, Li S, Higgs EF, Cabanov A, Wang X, Huang H et al. "Tumor heterogeneity and clonal cooperation influence the immune selection of IFN-gamma-signaling mutant cancer cells" *Nat Commun* 2020;11(1):602. 184.

[6] Cannas-Green D, Xie B, Huang J, Fan M, Wang A, Menaa C et al. "Dual blockade of CD47 and HER-2 eliminates radio resistant breast cancer cells" *Nat Commun* 2020;11(1):4591.

[7] Penter L, Dietze K, Bullinger L, Westermann J, Rahn HP, Hansmann L "FACS single cell index sorting is highly reliable and

determines immune phenotypes of clonally expanded T cells" *Eur J Immunol* 2018;48(7):1248-1250.

[8] Zebeck RM, De Jong E, Chin WL, Schuster IS, Fear VS, Casey TH et al. "Sensitization to immune checkpoint blockade through activation of a STAT1/NK axis in the tumor microenvironment" *Sci Transl Med* 2019;11(501);eaav7816.

[9] Dudley ME, Wunderlich JR, Robbins PF, Yang JC, Hwu P et al. "Cancer regression and autoimmunity in patients after clonal repopulation with anti-tumor lymphocytes" *Science* 2002;298(5594):850-4.

[10] Ucker DS, Levine JS "Exploitation of apoptotic regulation in cancer" *Front Immunol* 2018;9:241.

Chapter 16

SYSTEMS OF IMMUNE EVASION ARE INHERENT TO THE INFLAMMATORY RESPONSE TO TUMORIGENESIS

ABSTRACT

Abstract participation of cell injury and of an array of emerging damage-association antigen profiles is distributional in terms of a strictly incorporated series of dimensions that project as a paradoxical series of emerging immune evasion mechanisms. In such terms, incongruent redefinition of tumorigenesis is inherent participant within a process of immune evasion per se, as projected in terms of such distributional dynamics. Transport phenomena are derived dimensions as incorporated within specific contexts for further proliferation and spread of the malignant cells. The transformational modulators for such events arise as an inflammatory response, and as dictated paradoxically by the resulting series of immune evasion responses incorporated as proliferation and metastatic spread of the tumor cells.

INTRODUCTION

A paramount concept of pro-tumors is the intrinsically inherent component formulation of tumor-associated inflammation. In such terms, inflammation constitutes a component of emerging tumors in a manner that indicates the evolving dynamics of the carcinogenic phenomenon. To improve immunotherapy efficacy, targeting Wnt/Beta-catenin singling should be a high priority for combinatorial tumor therapy to reconstitute T cell response [1]. Inflammation comprises a whole series of systems that account for the establishment of the tumor and the evolving sustainment of progression of that tumor. The dynamic attributes of diverse CD45+ immune cells add new dimensions to the immune landscape of hepatocellular cancer [2]. It is within such a framework that immunogenesis and also immune escape arise as dys-homeostasis of the tumor microenvironment within the context of hierarchical development of a heterogeneous population of emerging tumor cells.

Inflammation is closely related to immunity, the identical immune cell populations contributing to both inflammation and the immune response; prevalent myeloid derived suppressor cells, M2 polarised macrophages and Treg are found in pancreatic adenocarcinoma [3]. In terms beyond the simple editing process of the immune response, there develops a series of directional parameters carried forward by the tumor-inherent inflammation that constitutes tumor-effective modulation of the microenvironment.

TUMOR DEVELOPMENT

In developmental contexts of a given tumor, the emergence of substantial evolution of carcinogenesis both constitutes component formulation of the inflammatory milieu and also a means of immune responsiveness within contexts for further tumorigenesis. As a mediator of immune surveillance and host defence TRAIL cytokines combine with death receptors to initiate a cascade of apoptotic events [4]. It is the realized dimension for inflammation to constitute intrinsic and multiple mechanisms within systems biology of carcinogenesis.

Natural Killer cells are regulatory cells implicated in reciprocal interactions with dendritic cells, T cells, macrophages and endothelial cells [5]. The derivative nature of tumor formulation, hence, is inherent to the potential for an antitumor immune response. In principle, tumor evolution can be controlled by cytotoxic innate and adaptive immune cells [6]. Substantial derivation of the inflammatory milieu of a given tumor incorporates opposing dimensions, and also formulations for an inherent attribute for tumor escape derived from the immuneosurveillance mechanics of the tumor micro-environment.

Tumor-Associated Inflammation

Metastases are systems for appraisal of the tumor-associated inflammation within the context of a variable immune response. Cyclooxygenase activity appears as a driver of immune suppression across species and its inhibition energises with anti-PD-1 blockade in eradication of tumors [7].

The evolutionary adaptation of tumorigenesis, in the face of an emerging and potential immune response, incorporates redefining terms that issue directional attributes of a conversion of mild inflammation to a harsh inflammatory tumor milieu. Several immune protumor effector mechanisms up regulate chronic inflammation and thus altering the balance between protumor and antitumor immunity [8]. The substantial presence of tumor-associated inflammation hence dominates the dynamics of tumorigenesis that is projected as evasion from immunosurveillance. The development of tumor- associated inflammation accounts for a novel incorporation of systems of immunogenicity and also for tumor-induced immune evasion. Ambiguity exists in research findings regarding the role of immune cells in modulating the metastatic microenvironment and determining cancer cell fate [9]. The distributional dynamics of such constitutive inflammation redefines the contextual derivation of much of the tumor attributes within the complex projection of such inflammatory reactivities.

Tumorigenesis

The constitutive derivation of inflammation inherent to tumorigenesis evolves, in redefining terms, the system biology of a process-carcinogenesis that is carried forward as tumor establishment and also as metastatic potential for further growth and spread of the tumor cells.

This is well illustrated by angiogenesis as an intrinsic attribute of tumorigenesis within the system profile for spread of the neoplasm. The redefining indices for such developmental dynamics is profile modulation of a tumor that, from the moment of inception, is modulated by an inflammatory response both in terms of ongoing damage-associated antigen recognition and as also response to further tumor growth. Adoptive cell therapy with tumor infiltrating lymphocytes induces objective tumor regression in many types of cancer including melanoma, cholangiocarcinoma and cervical squamous cell carcinoma [10]. The emergence of system dynamics hence incorporates the cytokine and chemokine derivations of tissue injury intrinsically incorporated within the tumor-associated inflammatory series of modulating responses.

Macrophage related genes play a central role in the modulation of the immune microenvironment in many human cancers [11].

System Profiles

System profiles are projections of a second-organ nature of the tumorigenesis as incorporated within redefinitions of biology of transformation of injured cells. The incorporation of an inflammatory response is defining terms of the carcinogenesis phenomenon as portrayed by the emergence of immunotolerance. In such terms, ongoing derivation of malignant transformation is simple formulation of a multitude of inflammatory responses that partake to the emerging immune escape of the tumor cells.

Such formulations are hence definitive expressions of carcinogenesis in terms of the context of subsequent metastatic spread of the malignant cells.

Directional Motivation

Directional motivation of tumor-associated inflammation can potentially account for immune tolerance within the system formulations that distribute profiles of congruence of the immune escape of individual and also of group biology of the emerging tumor cells. In such terms, the proliferation of tumor cells is inherently incorporated within relative dimensions for further tumor cell proliferation.

Conclusion

The performance dynamics of inflammation and of an effective immune response demonstrate the attributes for further proliferation and spread of the tumor cells, as categorically defined by the systems of enhanced tumor and immune responsiveness. In such terms, the populations of tumor cells are illustrative dynamics of an immune response that paradoxically redefines the carcinogenesis process as simple juxtapositioning of biologic dyshomeostasis mechanisms.

Such dys-functionalities are the sustainment of attributes for further growth and spread of the tumor within appraisal recognition of inflammation as modulator-dysfunction of the immune response. Component reappraisal of inflammation is therefore the hallmark of systems of immune recognition of tumor cells. The system incorporation of inflammation and of immune evasion hence is biology of a dysfunction as projected within profile dynamics for the recognition of damage-associated antigen profiles. The redistribution of cytokine and chemokine responses is simply consequences of an inflammatory responsiveness within the substantial reappraisal of system biology of cell derivation and modulation of cell spread. In such terms, inflammation directly incorporates modulation of the immune response that strictly re-categorizes the immune responsiveness.

REFERENCES

[1] Li X, Xiang Y, Li F, Yin C, Li B, Ke X "WNT/beta-catenin signaling pathway regulating T cell-inflammation in the tumor microenvironment" *Front Immunol* 2019;10:2293.

[2] Zhang Q, He Y, Luo N, Patel SJ, Han Y, Gao R et al. "Landscape and dynamics of single immune cells in hepatocellular carcinoma" *Cell* 2019;179(4):829-845.

[3] Padoan A, Plebani M, Basso D "Inflammation and pancreatic cancer: focus on metabolism, cytokines, and immunity" *Int J Mol* 2019;20(3):676.

[4] Khandia R, Munjal A "Interplay between inflammation and cancer" *Adv Protein Chem Struct Biol* 2020;119:119-245.

[5] Vivier E, Tomasello E, Baratin M, Walzer T, Ugolini S "Functions of natural killer cells" *Nat Immunol* 2008;9(5):402-10.

[6] Gonzalez H, Hagerling C, Werb Z "Roles of the immune system in cancer: from tutor initiation to metastatic progression" *Genes Dev* 2018;32(19-20):1267-1284.

[7] Zelenay S, van der Veen AG, Boettcher JP, Snelgrove KJ, Rogers N, Acton SE et al. "Cyclooxygenase-dependent tumor growth through evasion of immunity" *Cell* 2015;162(6):1257-70.

[8] Ostrand-Rosenberg S "Immune surveillance: a balance between protumor and antitumor immunity" *Curr Opin Genet Dev* 2008;18(1):11-8.

[9] Gonzalez H, Robles I, Werb Z "Innate and acquired immune surveillance in the post dissemination phase of metastasis" *FEBS J* 2018;285(4):654-664.

[10] Kumar A, Watkins R, Vilhelm AE "Cell therapy with TILs: training and taming T cells to fight cancer" *Front Immunol* 2021;12:690499.

[11] Chen Y, Zhang C, Zou X, Yu M, Yang B, Ji CF et al. "Identification of macrophage related gene in colorectal cancer patients and their functional roles" *BMC Med Genomics* 2021;14(1):159.

Chapter 17

Heterogeneous Dendritic Cell Subset Interchange as Tumor Immunosuppression

Abstract

Systems of turnover of DC subsets are primary modulators of the tumor microenvironmentally induced immunosuppression as further conferred within the contextually evolving pathways of various cytokines and VEGF. Tumor cell expansion is expression of such DC subset interchange that further involves dimensions for growth and expansion of the tumor lesion. Participation of the high levels of heterogeneity of DC subsets discloses the attributes of induction and modulation that dynamically provide inherent participation of the immunosuppression that pervades the tumor microenvironment. In terms beyond direct modulation, the autocrine systems of VEGF production and action are expressive dynamics for the evolution of systems of cooperative interface as dictated by VEGF action.

INTRODUCTION

An autocrine functionality of angiogenic factors such as Vascular Endothelial Growth Factor (VEGF) production by dendritic cells (DC) performs central axial series of modulatory actions within the complex performance of antigen presentation by these DC. With regard to such functionality, myeloid DC associated with the tumor microenvironment perform transitional shifts in phenotype and immunologic profiles that enhance the evolutionary course of many tumor types. Monocytes are a heterogeneous system with functions of both pro- and antitumor immunity, including differentiation into DC [1]. In terms, therefore, of such functionality, VEGF proves a biomarker in the demarcation of a series of transformational steps aimed ultimately to the creation of immunosuppression of the tumor microenvironment. Tumor infiltrating myeloid cells, including DC, monocytes and macrophages, are key regulators of cancer lesion progression [2]. The monocyte subset of myeloid-derived suppressor cells are highly plastic and their differentiation to DC and macrophages is determined largely by the tumor microenvironment [3].

In the development of an angiogenic or VEGF milieu, the DC evolve as modulators in terms of a vasculogenic environment that is conducive towards the transformational evolution of myeloid and also plasmacytoid DC, towards tolerance, and in the context of antigen presentation.

The potent capability of DC to initiate and regulate adaptive immune systems underpins the generation of anti-tumor immune reactivity [4]. Classical DC comprises two subsets, cDC1 and cDC2, based on phenotype markers and ability to prime CD8 and CD4 T cells [5]. The further promotional dynamics of tolerance are simply a dysfunctional attribute, also, of VEGF in terms that enhance effects of expansion of regulatory T immune cells. The relative dimensions borne out by the increments of dissociation and reactive actions of DC-related tumor microenvironment indicate the plastic modulatory microenvironment that primarily responds to angiogenic autocrine systems affecting DC.

Immunosuppression

The proportionality in evolution of substantial increment in immunosuppression that accompanies VEGF production and action indicates the performance dynamics of tumor growth and tumor cell expansion as dictated by shifts in transition of immature and mature DC as further proposed by the tolerant modulatory roles of reduction of co-stimulatory factors. The chemokine axis of migratory dimensions proposes further modulation of a potential antitumor immune response, as modified amplification in expansion of the tumor cells, and as borne out by immature dendritic cell dominance that participates with the vasculogenic response within the tumor microenvironment.

Tumor Cell Proliferation

The proliferative indices of performance dynamics of the tumor cell production of a tolerogenic microenvironment are hence representation of the plasticity of the DC, as projected within systems for further expansion of the tumor cells.

Single-cell gene expression investigations have shown widespread reprogramming across multiple cellular elements in the gastric cancer microenvironment in terms of a heterogenous cellular milieu [6]. The developmental attributes for emergence of DC plasticity are inherent differential modulation of various inflammatory cytokines and also as a shift from the Th1 to Th2 phenotype of the lymphocytes. Mass cytometry or complete transcriptome sequencing of a cell population or at an individual cell level have unveiled previously unknown populations of DC [7]. In such terms, the incremental attributes of tumor cell pools are associated, in closely related modes of participation of the DC populations, with highly heterogeneous immunophenotype expression, in a realization dimension that proves effective as tolerogenic immune response. Whether monocyte-derived DC are superior over other DC subsets is unknown, and promoting anti-tumor immune responses likely depends on tumor type and the constitution of the tumor microenvironment [8].

Immune Tolerance

The cooperative actions for immune tolerance indicate that VEGF production and action include the emergence of both sprouting vessels and also the generation of endothelial cells from blood-borne myeloid DC, as conveyed by the dynamics of a further enhanced tolerogenic and immunosuppressive tumor microenvironment. It is in terms of such scenario that the distributional phenomena govern the dynamic turnover of proliferating tumor cell pools, as these enhance the immunosuppression exerted by the tumor microenvironment. Modulatory mechanisms of the tumor microenvironment include effects on function of myeloid populations, recruitment and survival of myeloid subsets, and the functional reprogramming or activation of these cells [9]. The significant modulatory roles, as exerted on the DC, are further indices of turnover of the DC themselves, as these in turn contribute in multimodal fashion to the immunosuppression.

VEGF Action and Autocrine Systems

It is, in such terms, that the tumor cell proliferation and turnover include the formulation of VEGF production and action, as envisaged by dimensions of DC participation, as conveyed by systems of induced modulation of pre-existing tumor vessels, and of the generation of endothelial cell like populations that perform incremental modulation of the DC.

DC or monocyte-like cells contribute to angiogenic agent action, as dictated by evidential involvement of systems, in recognition of proinflammatory cytokines, and of antigens that are being processed by the DC. The inclusion of system profiles of increment of immunosuppressive effect within the tumor microenvironment constitutes actual terms of reference of VEGF production by the DC. The dynamics of involvement, as carried forward by DC participation, allow for the emergence of DC autocrine systems for further modulation of the tumor microenvironment. Context induces diversification of monocytes and neutrophil myeloid cells in modulating and orchestrating response of the tumor microenvironment [10].

System profile of DC modulation of immune response appears an autocrine performance as dictated by the DC subsets themselves. In the realization of interaction between DC subsets, it is evident that heterogeneity of DC subsets includes both killer subsets and tolerogenic DC, as projected by pathways of evolutionary response, on the one hand, and of the production of angiogenic agents. Myeloid cells hence have been proposed as therapeutic targets in solid cancer lesions [11]. Development of therapeutic approaches to deplete or reprogram myeloid cells in tumors is an emerging field of interest [12, 13].

The incremental dynamics of the tumor microenvironmental immunosuppression allow for the emergence of multi-modal DC and tumor cell interaction that, descriptively, is expressed in terms of an interchange of mature DC, on the one hand, and of immature DC on the other.

SYSTEM PROFILES OF DENDRITIC CELLS

In such terms, the performed attributes of antigen capture and of the modulated capacity for antigen processing and presentation by DC, are systems of expression that convey directly and indirectly to expansion of the tumor cell pools, as systems of transitional biology of the DC. Indeed, further modulation of the immunosuppressive tumor environment is inherent dimension of the primacy of the DC biology of progression within the milieu of re-characterization of immune response to tolerogenicity.

Conclusion

Performance interchange between a multitude of DC subsets is inherent manifestation of a projected dimension of cooperative DC participation that is actively evolving to a tolerogenic tumor microenvironment. Subset DC dominance, in turn, modulates the tumor cells as expressive index of performance, as dictated within the milieu context of the tumor cell pools and the tumor microenvironment.

It is in terms of DC subset interchange that the contextual participation of tumor cell expansion includes, in particular, the autocrine actions of VEGF that is produced by DC, and also projected by the induced immunosuppression. VEGF is itself immunosuppressive, as derived from increments of tumor cell hypoxia within the expanded lesion that formulates multi-modal involvement of autocrine systems of VEGF generation and induced immune modulation.

References

[1] Olingy CE, Dinh HQ, Hedrick CC "Monocyte heterogeneity and functions in cancer" *J Leukoc Biol* 2019;106(2):309-322.

[2] Zilionis R, Engblom C, Pfirschke C, Savova V, Zemmour D, Saatcioglu HD et al. "Single-cell transcriptomics of human and mouse lung cancers reveals conserved myeloid populations across individuals and species" *Immunity* 2019;50(5):1317-1334.

[3] Tcyganov E, Mastio J, Chen E, Gabrilovich DI "Plasticity of myeloid-derived suppressor cells in cancer" *Curr Opin Immunol* 2018;51:76-82.

[4] Lee YS, Radford KJ "The role of dendritic cells in cancer" *Int Rev Cell Mol Biol* 2019;348:123-178.

[5] Brown CC, Gudjonson H, Pritykin Y, Deep D, Lavallee VP, Mendoza A et al. "Transcriptional basis of mouse and human dendritic cell heterogeneity" *Cell* 2019;179:846-863.

[6] Sathe A, Grimes SM, Lau BT, Chen J, Suarez C, Huang RJ et al. "Single-cell genomic characterisation reveals the cellular reprogramming of the gastric tumor microenvironment" *Clin Cancer Res* 2020;26(11):2640-2653.

[7] Hubert M, Gobbini E, Bendriss-Vermare N, Caux C, Valladeau-Guilemond J "Human tumor-infiltrating dendritic cells: from in situ visualisation to high-dimensional analyses" *Cancers* (Basel) 2019;11(8):1082.

[8] Huber A, Dammeijer F, Aerts JGJV, Vroman H "Current state of dendritic cell-based immunotherapy: opportunities for *in vitro* antigen loading of different DC subsets?" *Front Immunol.* 2018;9:2804.

[9] Janicova A, Becker N, Xu B, Wutzler S, Vollrath JT, Hildebrand F, Ehnert S et al. "Tuning the tumor myeloid microenvironment to fight cancer" *Front Immunol* 2019;10:1611.

[10] Jeong J, Suh Y, Jung K "Context drives diversification of monocytes and neutrophils in orchestrating the tumor microenvironment" *Front Immunol* 2019;10:1817.

[11] Cotechini T, Medler TR, Coussens LM "Myeloid cells as targets for therapy in solid tumors" *Cancer J* 2015;21(4):343-50.

[12] Kiss M, Van Gassen S, Movahedi K, Saeys Y, Laoui D "Myeloid cell heterogeneity in cancer: not a single cell alike" *Cell Immunol* 2018;330:188-201.

[13] Clappaert EJ, Murgaski A, Van Damme H, Kiss M, Laoui D "Diamonds in the rough: harnessing tumor-associated myeloid cells for cancer therapy" *Front Immunol* 2018;9:2250.

Chapter 18

Recurrent Immune Responses Are Primary Reactivity to the Tumor Microenvironment Rather Than to the Integral Tumor Cells Themselves

Abstract

Participation parameters of antigen specificity are response elements of persistent turnover of the dendritic cells and of the T lymphocyte subsets, as borne out by the incremental dimensions for integral microenvironment dynamics. In a real sense, the primary target for DC and immune response is constituted by the tumor microenvironment rather than by the tumor cells or of the tumor lesion itself. It is in such terms that the tumor microenvironment constitutes the primary target of the antitumor response as verified by the intense dynamics of this tumor microenvironment. The pathways induced by such targeting of the microenvironment potentially prevent immune response to most of the tumor lesion in terms of ongoing modulation and remodeling.

It is significant to view the primal and repeated immune responsiveness to tumors as a characterized series of cascade events overwhelmingly targeting the tumor microenvironment rather than directly to the integral tumor cells themselves.

INTRODUCTION

The potentiality for targeting of tumor cells with dendritic cells (DC) depends, to a large extent, on the different modalities that govern trafficking of the DC and other immune cells. Modulation of the microenvironmental components can help control tumorigenesis [1]. In large measure, the differential abilities to produce an efficient antitumor effect involve the evolution of DC within the scopes for preservation of DC from such processes as apoptosis. The incumbent dysfunctionality of the various chemokines is a central issue in the development and maintenance of antitumor effect. Growing evidence indicates that the innate immune cells as well as adaptive immune cells contribute to cancer progression [2].

In addition, in particular, the trapping of DC within the tumor lesion calls for the modulation of the tumor environment as indeed controlled by matrix metalloproteinases and the tissue inhibitors of such matrix proteases.

IMMUNE CELL HOMING

The governance for the homing of peripheral DC to tumor, and their subsequent trafficking to regional lymph nodes, is integral to the mobilization of the loaded DC to the T cell-rich regions of the draining lymph nodes. Most tutor cells express antigens that can be recognised by host CD8(+) T cells and evasion of these cells allows for progressive cancer growth [3].

Cross-priming, where DC activate CD8 T cells by cross-presenting exogenous antigens, is critical to the generation of anti-timor CD8 T cell immunity [4].

Also, the evolutionary course of the activated T lymphocytes is beset by dynamics of imbalance as projected by systems of action of a wide variety of immune cells such as Natural Killer Cells, Langerhans cells and also B lymphocytes.

Such realization of cell recruitment is a generic phenomenon of DC susceptibility to various arrays of chemokines and of chemokine receptors. The recent discovery of immune "checkpoints" that suppress immune activity and avoid auto-immunity has permitted enhancement in reactivity to cancer cells [5].

PROGRAMS OF DC MOBILITY

The substantiality of such considerations indicates the reformulation of programs of mobility of DC, as dictated by the internal milieu of tumors, and also by expression programs that tend to integrate the immune antitumor response. In such terms, the generalized immune trafficking modalities induce the realization of a systemic involvement that globally participates within systematic localization of the DC within the tumor lesion. In large measure, the actuation of the immune response involves the creation of a series of cascade pathways that induce the initiation and maintenance of the antitumor responsiveness, as brought forward by participation and conversion of immature DC to mature DC.

It is further to such considerations that the involvement of dynamics of trafficking of a whole range of immune cells is permissive phenomenon in its own right, as indeed reformulated and continuously reformulated.

Dynamics of the attributes for migration of DC is hence a working model for the mobility of T lymphocytes that are virtual targets for the mobile DC in terms of activation or priming of the T cells, or for cytotoxic T cells. Precise and accurate predictive biomarkers can potentially be identified forpersonalzed immunotherapy clinically [6]. In a real sense, the evolutionary dynamics for further spread of the DC and lymphocytes are integral to an induction for further immune targeting of the tumor cells, as portrayed by memory immune cells. Memory T cells are central players in the case of recurrent tumors, within simple considerations of reactivation of both DC and T lymphocytes.

Tumors arise within a context of an *in vivo* cancer environment that is both cause and consequent of carcinogenesis, resulting in de-evolution via indirect and direct cellular interactivity [7].

In such measure the incremental dynamics of induction of DC and T lymphocytes are transformed to activation within the milieu of the tumor microenvironment.

It is the realization of cell injury, and of apoptosis and necrosis of tumor cells, that offers the opportunity to enhance and render robust the immune response. Chemoimmunotherapy appears to activate a strong T cell antitumor immune response by inducing immunogenic cell death and this has prompted a number of clinical trials [8]. It is within a contextual dynamics for spread mobility that the DC prove potent mechanisms in the realization of antitumor cell susceptibility to ongoing transformation of the tumor microenvironment. The actual participation of a multi-cascade series of enhancing events allows for the emergence for further antitumor processes leading to a potential increment in clinical regression of the tumor. NK cells induce recruitment of conventional DC1 into the tumor microenvironment thus enhancing cancer immune control [9]. It is within such systems of response that the immune cells offer a series of recurrent pathways of targeting of the tumor cells and of the tumor microenvironment.

Responsiveness

Distinguishing the effective responsiveness allows for the emergence of tumor cell survival as portrayed by dynamics of expansion of DC and of T cells as sufficiently robust immune responses; these mainly occur repeatedly and also through processing and presentation dynamics by integral groups of heterogeneous subsets of DC cells.

In terms of ongoing participation of cell injury within tumors, the ongoing involvement of pathways for constitutive reappraisal of tumor cell antigenicity allows for the realization of a repertoire for repeated immune response targeting of the tumor cells. Increasing evidence suggests that the DC systems display a wide range of dysfunctional states in the tumor microenvironment and that these impair antitumor immune response [10].

Dynamics of Replay

Dynamics of replay of the immune response appear to implicate a fine tuning of the antitumor reactivity series of events within a context of memory T cell reactivation.

In such measure, the incremental potential for antitumor immune response bespeaks of a series of immunologically motivated series of trafficking modalities within encompasses of parallel events of reactivity. p53 dysfunction in various cellular compartments of the tumor microenvironment promotes immunosuppression and immune evasion [11]. The immune systems are both passive and reactive pathways for induced participation of the tumor cell targeting events, as further projected by tumor cell apoptosis and necrosis. It is such incremental dynamics that provokes waves of immune response, and the evolution participation of pathways for renewal and remodulation of the antitumor cell targeting and response.

Conclusion

Provocative response on the part of the immune system is reformulated by DC as provided by dynamics of antigen detection, and also by such systems as tumor cell expansion and turnover.

In the creation of such antitumor immune response, the derivation phenomena of the DC and T lymphocyte reactivities are ongoing repetition of cascade pathway response, as indeed illustrated by functional and dysfunctional attributes of memory T cells, and as further projected by remodulation series of events by the tumor microenvironment.

It is in terms of incremental response, and further response, that the tumor microenvironment encompasses a series of specific and patterned responses, that eventually confirm the attributes of the tumor lesion. This grows and expands within a suppressive tumor microenvironment. The system pathways of DC response are series reformulations that adhere to such pathways as high endothelial cell systems of afferent lymphatics and of intranodal homing of the dendritic cells to T cell-rich regions, thus participating in systems of recognition response to tumor cell antigenicity.

It is, therefore, within the trafficking modality choice for DC homing to the tumor and to the tumor microenvironment, that systems of repetitive cascades of response potentially integrate pathways of reactivation of T lymphocytes as terms of reference of the antigen specificity of these cells and of DC.

References

[1] Arneth B "Tumor microenvironment" *Medicina* (Kaunas) 2019;56(1):15.

[2] Henshaw DC, Shevde LA "The tumor microenvironment innately modulates cancer progression" *Cancer Res* 2019;79(18):4557-4566.

[3] Gajewski TF, Schreiber H, Fu YX "Innate and adaptive immune cells in the tumor microenvironment" *Nat Immunol* 2013;14(10):1014-22.

[4] Fu C, Jiang A "Dendritic cells and CD8 T cell immunity in tumor microenvironment" *Front Immunol* 2018;9:3059.

[5] Frankel T, Lanfranca MP, Zou W "The role of tumor microenvironment in cancer immunotherapy" *Adv Exp Med Biol* 2017;1036:51-64.

[6] Baba Y, Nomoto D, Okadome K, Ishimoto T, Iwatsuki M, Minamoto Y et al. "Tumor immune microenvironment and immune checkpoint inhibitors in oesophageal squamous cell carcinoma" *Cancer Sci* 2020;111(9):3132-3141.

[7] Casey SC, Amedei A, Aquilano K, Azmi AS, Benencia F, Bhakta D et al. "Cancer prevention and therapy through the modulation of the tumor microenvironment" *Semin Cancer Biol* 2015;35 Suppl (Suppl):S199-223.

[8] Zhou F, Feng B, Yu H, Wang D, Wang T, Ma Y et al. "Tumor microenvironment-activatable prodrug vesicles for nano enabled cancer chemoimmunotherapy combining immunogenic cell death induction and CD47 blockade" *Adv Mater* 2019;31(14):e1805888.

[9] Bottcher JP, Bonavita E, Chakravarty P, Blees H, Cabeza-Cabrerizo M, Sammicheli S et al. "NK cells stimulate recruitment of cDC1 into the tumor microenvironment promoting cancer immune control" *Cell* 2018;172(5):1022-1037.

[10] Zhu S, Yang N, Wu J, Wang X, Wang W, Liu YJ et al. "Tumor microenvironment-related dendritic cell deficiency: a target to enhance tumor immunotherapy" *Pharmacy Res* 2020;259:103980.

[11] Cui Y, Guo G "Immunomodulatory function of the tumor suppressor p53 in ghost immune response and the tumor microenvironment" *Int J Mol Sci* 2016;17(11):1942.

Chapter 19

THE IMMUNOLOGIC NON-RESPONSE IS A PHYSIOLOGIC, CONDITIONAL AND HOMEOSTATIC STATE OF AN INTEGRAL IMMUNE SYSTEM TOWARDS TUMOR ANTIGENICITY

ABSTRACT

Evidential reformulation of the tumor-related immune non-response is integral to an immune system that is dominantly tolerant to foreign antigen and to tumor antigens. The descriptive participation of such tumor-related immune tolerant states is a paradoxical conditioning that establishes the immune non-response in terms of a dominant homeostatic state that operates to control the otherwise reactive immune system. It is significant to view the non-response of the immune system as central operative axis of the reactivities of DC and T lymphocytes to a progressing tumor lesion. In such realizing terms, the immune non-response is a highly plastic series of suppressive indices in the defined homeostatic attributes of a physiologic conditioning of the integral immune system.

Introduction

Dendritic cell (DC) states of immunologic tolerance are actively acquired polarization and conditioning responses that dominantly induce an immunosuppressive tumor microenvironment. Tumor exosomes inhibit the maturation and migration of DC and enhance the immune suppression of these immune cells [1]. The incremental dimensions of such tolerant states involve a broad array of procedural maneuvers in terms of the consistently projected involvement of dysfunctionality of DC and of reactive T-cell responses. The diverse functions of DC subsets are shaped by the tumor microenvironment [2]. In such setting, the DC dysfunctionalities are closely linked to the activation of T cells that are present in the tumor microenvironment.

Dendritic and T-Cell Cooperativity

The close cooperative dimensions of DC and T cells are incumbent parametric coordinates within the evolutionarily established non-response of the immune system to foreign antigens and to tumor antigens.

The innate immune memory is a powerful targeting framework to regulate immune homeostasis, priming and tolerance [3]. In such terms, the provocative increments of DC that constitute the early immune responses to tumor antigen incorporation of the actively acquired immune suppression, within the established milieu of immune senescence.

It is within the strictly evolving context of such reproducibility that immune senescence is constitutively conditioning, as proposed particularly by the immature DC. Tumor-infiltrating DC may also be implicated in tumor pathogenesis [4]. It is such contextualization of the DC dysfunctionalities that accounts for the overall dimensions of the immune non-response that involves the emergence of reduced costimulatory molecules and for the reinforcement of DC polarization. The significant contexts for immune suppression, as specific forms of immune senescence, evolve as descriptive and dynamic integers in inducing further immunosuppression. Macrophages, granulocytes and DC are essential myeloid cells for the function of both innate and adaptive immune responses [5].

IMMUNE SUPPRESSION VERSUS NON-RESPONSE

Apoptosis of T lymphocyte subsets and the active recruitment of suppressor T cells coordinately involve, in projected manner, the dimensions of immunosuppression that further the evolution of the tumor microenvironment. Such microenvironment is replete with the ongoing senescence effectors of the immune response, as further proposed by substantial depletion of the DC. The development of cooperative suppression is a dominant dimension, as proposed by tolerant DC subsets, within the context for reproducible DC depletion and dysfunctionality.

The proposed application of injury to DC is performance enforcement of positive effects that dominantly implicate the emergence of indoleamine 2,3 dioxygenase (IDO) DC in terms of immuno-suppression and immuno-senescence. DC have become the natural agents for antigen delivery [6]. The evolutionary characterization of the suppressive tumor microenvironment is constitutive emergence of such parameters as apoptosis and the loss of cell contact between DC and T lymphocytes, that dominantly suppress the immune response.

In clear and actual provisions for such immune dysfunctionalities, the further projection of myeloid and plasmacytoid DC incorporate also a polarization to a Type 1 T-cell response that may accompany conditioned immunosenescence. DC link the innate immune system to the adaptive response to initiate antigen-specific immune responses [7].

IMMUNO-SENESCENCE

A parent series of consequences of immunosenescence include, in particular, the shaping of an immunologically tolerant state that is generated primarily within the tumor core, with added the realization of depleted subsets of reactive DC components. Fibroblast heterogeneity is also implicated in microenvironmental immunosuppression [8]. The evolutionary process of tumor progression is further enhanced as remodulation of the tumor microenvironment, as proposed projection of apoptosis of T-lymphocyte subsets.

The concomitant emergence of both DC- and lymphocyte-suppression is performance dynamics that recharacterize the tolerance status of the tumor microenvironment. To enhance the efficacy of DC-based immunotherapy, a combination of treatments is essential [9]. Recharacterization of DC is a dysfunctional attribute in terms of ongoing pathways of pronounced suppression that, generically, shapes the immunosurveillance capacity by an otherwise potent immune response.

IMMUNE TOLERANCE

Cooperative dimensions operate in terms of immunologic tolerance in terms of a progressive tumor cell proliferation and spread, in terms of ongoing participation of the immunosenescence series of non-response states. Post-translational signatures such as glycans are key molecules implicated in the regulation of immunity versus tolerance [10]. The attributes for the interacting DC phenomena are participant increments of dimensionalized pathways for tumor progression.

The immunologic outcome depends on the state of DC activation [11]. The actualization of active participation of non-response of the immune system is itself dominant reactivity that proposes immuno-senescence.

Such a process involves therefore fundamental reshaping of the tumor microenvironment in suppressing DC- and T-lymphocyte reactivities. The immune system simultaneously mounts a response while tolerating self; many mechanisms of tolerance indeed are antigen non-specific [12].

DOMINANCE OF IMMUNE NON-RESPONSE

Paramount considerations of a series of non-responses, in terms of dominance of an immune non-response is central tenet within the evolutionary reshaping of the immune response and of the immune system as integral participation for further immune suppression. The result of an immune response is determined by the context exhibited by the acquired antigen, and also by the specific DC subsets implicated [13].

The diagnostic significance for an actively acquired immunologically tolerant state is central operative axis within such an immunity participation, as indeed provoked by the emergence of the suppressive tumor microenvironment. Most malignant lesions occur in the elderly and the immune suppressed, thus implicating an essential role for the cancer immune surveillance systems [14].

The integral immune system therefore operates dominantly in terms of an immune non-response, in the first instance, that, in evolutionary terms, allows for tolerance states of immune non-response. Some anticancer therapies may reverse tumor-mediated responses *in vivo*, as seen with 5-Fluorouracil [15]. The incremental involvement of functional dominance, as a parametric homeostatic reshaping of the tolerant immune response, allows for the further cooperative dimensions of physiologic adaptation of the primary responses of DC and T lymphocytes to tumor progression.

PHYSIOLOGIC HOMEOSTASIS OF IMMUNE NON-RESPONSE

Malignant lesions are not immunologically silent by evolve and react in a continuous bi-directional manner with the host immune system [16]. In terms, therefore, that bespeak of physiologic homeostasis, the immune non-response to primary tumor antigens is inherent re-characterization of the immune system as dimensionalized within systems that otherwise would induce plasticity of immune responsiveness. The innate immune memory is a biologic response that implicates epigenetic and metabolic reprogramming as trained immunity [17]. Therefore, in the realization of tumor-cell growth and spread, the related immune system evolution is primal dimension of a dominant immune non-response. Physiologic participation of injury to DC and T lymphocytes is added dimension within a global immune system that tolerates the emergence of tumor-cell progression.

CONCLUSION

The tolerant state of the immune non-response is a cardinal attribute of the global and integral immune system that further participates in the development of a suppressive tumor microenvironment.

The physiologic homeostatic conditioning of a primal immune response is integral to an immune system that dominates the shaped coordinates of an otherwise potent immune response to tumor antigens. In such terms, the ongoing participation of immune non-response is further projected as terms for the emergence of a series of evolutionary indices for immune suppression and for immuno-senescence. The derivative reformulations incriminate the substantial cooperative dominance of immune non-responses as paradoxical contexts for physiologic functional and dysfunctional attributes that go beyond simple immune responsiveness.

REFERENCES

[1] Ning Y, Shen K, Wu Q, Sun X, Bai Y, Xie Y et al. "Tumor exosomes block dendritic cells maturation to decrease the T cell immune response" *Immunol Lett* 2018;199:36-43.

[2] Wculek SK, Cueto FJ, Mujal AM, Melero I, Krummel MF, Sancho D "Dendritic cells in cancer immunology and immunotherapy" *Nat Rev Immunol* 2020;20(1):7-24.

[3] Mulder WJM, Ochando J, Joosten LAB, Fayad ZA, Netea MG "Therapeutic targeting of trained immunity" *Nat Rev Drug Discov* 2019;18(7):553-566.

[4] Tran Banco JM, Lamichhane P, Karyampudi L, Knutson KL "Tumor-infiltrating dendritic cells in cancer pathogenesis" *J Immunol* 2015;194(7):2095-91.

[5] Gabrilovich DI, Ostrand-Rosenberg S, Bronte V "Coordinated regulation of myeloid cells by tumors" *Nat Rev Immunol* 2012;12(4):253-68.

[6] Palucka K, Banchereau J "Cancer immunotherapy via dendritic cells" *Nat Rev Cancer* 2012;12(4):265-77.

[7] Mellman I "Dendritic cells: master regulators of the immune response" *Cancer Immunol Res* 2013;1(3):145-9.

[8] Costa A, Kieffer Y, Scholer-Dahirel A, Pelon F, Bourachot B, Cardon M et al. "Fibroblast heterogeneity and immunosuppressive environment in human breast cancer" *Cancer Cell* 2018;33(3):463-479.

[9] Bol KF, Schreibelt G, Gerritsen WR, de Vries IJ, Figdor CG "Dendritic cell-based immunotherapy: state of the art and beyond" *Clin Cancer Res* 2016;22(8):1897-906.

[10] Lubbers J, Rodriguez E, van Kooyk Y "Modulation of immune tolerance via siglec-sialic acid interactions" *Front Immunol* 2018;9:2807.

[11] Adema GJ "Dendritic cells from bench to bedside and back" *Immunol Lett* 2009;122(2):128-30.

[12] Moore JR "The benefits of diversity: heterogeneous DC populations allow for both immunity and tolerance" *J Theor Biol* 2014;357:86-102.

[13] Delamarre L, Mellman I "Harnessing dendritic cells for immunotherapy" *Semin Immunol* 2011;23(1):2-11.

[14] Jackaman C, Nelson DJ *Are macrophages, myeloid derived suppressor cells and neutrophils mediators of local suppression in healthy and cancerous tissues in aging hosts?*

[15] Apetoh L, Vegran F, Ladoire S, Ghiringhelli F "Restoration of antitumor immunity through selective inhibition of myeloid derived suppressor cells by anticancer therapies" *Curr Mol Med* 2011;11(5):365-72.

[16] Senovilla L, Aranda F, Galluzzi L, Kroemer G "Impact of myeloid cells on the efficacy of anticancer chemotherapy" *Curr Opin Immunol* 2014;30:24-31.

[17] Netea MG, Dominguez-Andres J, Barreiro LB, Chavakis T, Divangahi M, Fuchs E et al. "Defining trained immunity and its role in health and disease" *Nat Rev Immunol* 2020;20(6):375-388.

Chapter 20

DENDRITIC CELL PLASTICITY AS HISTORY OF PERFORMANCE DYNAMICS

ABSTRACT

Potent antitumor immune responses are beset by the nature of given DC activation and maturation programs as realized by system profiles of remodeling of plasticity issues and as further characterized by performance history of the DC. The development of such projection is integral to the system derivation of injury to DC and as further defined and redefined by a microenvironment of modulated potential and system programs for attempted conformity of plastic DC. Redistribution dynamics of plastic DC promote a strong potentiality for contrast confrontation towards tumor neoantigenicity. The performance history realization is intricate expression of biology mechanics of the DC intracellular plasticity in the first instance.

INTRODUCTION

The compounding effects of differentiation and maturation processes as expounded by dendritic cells (DC) are integral to an antitumor immune response within the perpetuating influence of an extensive cytokine network. Cancer evolves within a context of restricted DC activity [1].

The intricate dynamics of an immune response lie within the potent possible evolution of the tolerance mechanisms that belie such antitumor immune response. DC uniquely induce naive T cell activation and also effector differentiation [2]. In such terms, the progression of tumor evolution incriminate the emergence of tolerogenic clones of T lymphocytes within expounding dynamics of tumor cell survival and spread as primarily exemplified by the nature of both innate and adaptive immunity.

System Profiles

DC as heterogeneous populations are central to initiating, directing and regulating adaptive immune responses in tumor immunosurveillance [3]. The system profiles of antigen processing machinery are an expression of a whole series of co-stimulatory molecular species within the further exponential expression of cytokines and chemokines. Altered DC function and differentiation are likely to be a most fundamental series of mechanisms by which neoplasms escape immune responses [4].

Natural regulatory T cells control self-tolerance and are exclusively committed to suppressive function under all microenvironmental contexts [5]. In such manner, proposal evidence is inherent to the further compounding influences as verified within the nature of an antitumor immune response that constitutes shifting plasticity of DC.

It is further to such parameters that the proportional skewing of T lymphocytes to a Th1 phenotype is beset by realized dynamics of system reassessment and as profile models predicting such skewing of the lymphocyte response.

PROPORTIONALITY

Actual proportionality of the antitumor immune response is a multifunctionality of DC as further derivable from pathway reconstitution of immature and partly mature DC. Significant defects in DC functions hold the strong potentiality of a tolerance phenomenon as projected within the encompassed potential also of migratory attributes of DC. Within reaffirmation of activation of DC there emerges the redistribution dynamics of realized reactivities of the immune response as further enhanced by antitumor immunity. Aberrant functions of proteoglycans and glycosaminoglycans contribute significantly to cancer stem cell phenotype and also therapeutic resistance [6].

System profiles of a potent immune response to emerging and evolving tumor cells define and further redefine the status of the immune response as predetermined by dynamics of maturation of DC. Maturation of these is inherent attribute of the subsequent activation mechanics within system component biology of the immune response. Tumor and dendritic cell plasticity supports or otherwise limits tumor progression and indeed induces an immunosuppressive switch to enhance further tumor evolution [7]. The descriptive embodiment of pathway non-conformity is pronounced expression that inherently incorporates the migratory biology of activated immune cells and of DC.

TOLERANCE

Particularly pronounced is the tolerance of an immune pathway reconstitution as derived from functionalities of the DC maturation program. Two opposing contexts affecting DC are the induction of a tolerogenic profile and a pro-inflammatory profile due to plasticity [8].

Derivative phenomena are hence descriptive anatomy of the activation of DC as further proposed by the maturation programs that arise as DC activation. In terms therefore of unique attributes of DC to a specific tumor antigen profile there emerges the projection phenomenon of the antitumor immune response.

Further descriptive dynamics implicate a dysfunctional profile of the activation of DC that infiltrates tumors and peritumoral stroma. Suppressor of cytokine signaling 1 functions as a "non-classical" checkpoint blocker and it modulates DC via mechanisms of generation, maturation, antigen presentation, costimulatory signaling and cytokine production [9]. Increments of potentiality are particularly dominated as models of realized contrast of the tumor antigens as these repeatedly propose potential tolerance. The compounding actions of system profiles are integral expression of the nature of a projection series of processes determining plasticity of DC.

The design of multifaceted vehicles, the choice of surface molecules to specifically target DC, and the choice of adjuvants to guide and sustain DC maturation are being pursued [10]. The incremental antitumor immune response hence fails as descriptive anatomy of intracellular transport dynamics within DC. Processing machinery is manipulated in a manner that highly characterizes the venue of contrasting conformity towards the tumor antigen processes that are partly expressed by the neoplastic cells.

Heterogeneity

Antigen presentation programs are derived from the incumbent heterogeneity of system realization that accounts for the failure of the immune response as evidenced by re-constitutive imbalance of the plastic DC biology. DC-T cell interaction is shaped by the state of DC maturation, the type of DC subset, the cytokine microenvironment and the tissue location [11].

The performance mechanics of the antitumor immune response is itself an inherent expression of derived identity of the maturation and activation phenomena that primarily characterize DC. In conformity to pathway modulation of antigen processing, the incremental progression of tumor cell proliferation and spread incorporates the performance of an immune response that paradoxically is tolerogenic. In such terms, the re-characterization of potentials for activation and migration of DC further compounds derivative recombination of antigen profiles as significantly accounted for by the DC programs of maturation.

ANTITUMOR IMMUNITY

Modulation and remodulation of the antitumor immune response is hindered in terms of system profile skewing that propose pro-inflammatory cytokines and chemokines.

Prior performance dynamics institute profile re-characterization as projected within the system dynamics of a specific immune pattern of expression.

The redistribution anomalies arising within DC are hence performance attributes that permit the emergence for further change that prolongs tolerance to tumor neoantigens.

Distribution of DC dysfunctionality is hence a resultant interplay within the evolving dynamics of activation and maturation processes of projected DC. DC act at the interface of immunity and peripheral tolerance [12]. The significant encompassed derivation of such realization questions the nature of an inherent and integral projection process that itself is associated with the emergence of tumor neoantigenicity. The complex interplay of antigen redistribution is realized as plasticity of the DC. Innovative combinatorial therapeutic strategies are being explored to normalise the immune DC function in the tumor microenvironment and synergistically promote DC function [13].

The performance history of the DC is active template for the emergence forces towards plastic conformity of tolerogenic clones of T lymphocytes and of DC response.

Conclusion

The defining terms of tolerance of DC biology is expression of a cellular dynamics that characterizes DC plasticity. The realization forces for compromise towards immune tolerance are inherent expression of a process of maturation of the DC within system profiles of modeled potentiality. Novel antigenicity is a descriptive annotation of the tumor cell biology in its own right and as further projection in terms of the nature of the tolerance to an immune response. The specific derivative biology of increment is quantitative expression in the realization of the future migration of DC to secondary lymphoid organs as proposed by the nature of projection effects of pro-inflammatory cytokines and chemokines. Redistribution dynamics are hence incorporated within antigen processes that are themselves defined by intracellular transport machinery of the DC.

References

[1] Fucikova J, Palova-Jezinkova L, Bartunkova J, Spisek R "Induction of tolerance and immunity by dendritic cells: mechanisms and clinical applications" *Front Immunol* 2019;10:2393.

[2] Patente TA, Pinho MP, Oliveira AA, Evangelista GCM, Bergami-Santos PC, Barbuto JAM "Human dendritic cells: their heterogeneity and clinical application potential in cancer immunotherapy" *Front Immunol* 2019;9:3176.

[3] Strioga M, Schijns V, Powell DJ Jr, Pasukoniene V, Dobrovolskiene N, Michalek J "Dendritic cells and their role in tumor immunosurveillance" *Innate Immun* 2013;19(1):98-111.

[4] Yang L, Carbone DP "Tumor-host immune interactions and dendritic cell dysfunction" *Adv Cancer Res* 2004;92:13-27.

[5] Schiavon V, Duchez S, Branchtein M, How-Kit A, Cassius C, Daunay A et al. "Microenvironment tailors nTreg structure and function" *Proc Natl Acad Sci USA* 2019/116(13):6298-6307.
[6] Vitale D, Kumar Katakam S, Greve B, Jang B, Oh ES, Alaniz L et al. "Proteoglycans and glycosaminoglycans as regulators of cancer stem cell function and therapeutic resistance" *FEBS J* 2019;286(15):2870-2882.
[7] Granot Z, Fridlender ZG "Plasticity beyond cancer cells and the 'immunosuppressive switch' " *Cancer Res* 2015;75(21):4441-5.
[8] Motta JM, Rumjanek VM "Sensitivity of dendritic cells to microenvironment signals" *J Immunol Res* 2016;2016:4753607.
[9] Ilangumaran S, Bobbala D, Ramanathan S "SOCS1: regulator of T cells in autoimmunity and cancer" *Curr Top Microbiol Immunol* 2017;410:159-189.
[10] Gornati L, Zenoni I, Granucci F "Dendritic cells in the cross hair for the generation of tailored vaccines" *Front Immunol* 2018;9:1484.
[11] Waisman A, Lukas D, Clausen BE, Yogev N "Dendritic cells as gatekeepers of tolerance" *Semin Immunopathol* 2017;39(2):153-163.
[12] Adema GJ "Dendritic cells from bench to bedside and back" *Immunol Lett* 2009/122(2):128-30.
[13] Galati D, Zanotta S "Empowering dendritic cell cancer vaccination: the role of combinatorial strategies" *Cytotherapy* 2018;20 (11):1309-1323.

Chapter 21

CONTACT MECHANICS OF IMMUNE EVASION INVOLVE SUPPRESSION OF THE ANTIGEN-PRESENTATION STEP AND OF THE TUMOR-MIRRORED MIGRATION OF THE DENDRITIC CELLS

ABSTRACT

Intense dynamics of migrating dendritic cells dominate the mechanics of priming of the T lymphocytes in draining lymph nodes and spleen. The process of maturation of the dendritic cells is incumbent phenomenon of a cytokine profile secretion and also of the antigen-presentation interacting with systems of induction and modulation of tumor neoantigenicity. The system profile, as induced series of reactivities, is permissive contact processing of the DC presentation of tumor neoantigens.

The tumor microenvironment is system profile for such induction, as further compounded by migration of the antigen-loaded DC. The aberrant systems of cellular confrontation account for an induction phenomenon that converges as modulation of the tumor neoantigenicity and of a suppressive tumor microenvironment.

Introduction

The investigative aspects of both hormonal and autonomic nervous systems involve aspects of dendritic cells (DC) that process and present antigens to antigen-specific T lymphocytes. In such terms, glucocorticoids tend to suppress antigen-presentation by DC cells. It is further to such considerations that a network series of mechanisms operates in a manner to suppress immune response to tumor antigens. Resident memory T cells are crucial to tumor immunology; close contact with tumor cells, dominant expression of checkpoint receptors and recognition of cancer cells may enhance action of immune checkpoint inhibitors [1].

It is significant to consider the optional series of patterns of response to tumor cells as further mechanistic response-contact with T lymphocytes. The broad range of responsiveness of DC, in particular, dominates the process of maturation of DC towards the suppression of proliferation and of spread of the T lymphocytes.

Immune Response

The mandatory immune response to foreign antigen is largely recapitulated in the immune responsiveness to tumor neoantigens. The dynamic and evolving cross-talk between inflammatory and cancer cells appears to be direct and contact-dependent, but is also conveyed by soluble and exosome-carried cytokines [2].

In such manner, the evolving substantiality of the derived immune escape of tumor cells includes the reactivities evoked by contact dynamics of DC with primed T lymphocytes, and also with regard to essentially naïve lymphocytes.

Besides direct cell-to-cell contact, extracellular vesicles add a new layer of complexity to the modulation of immune responses [3]. The proportionality of such phenomena is projected as system preference modules in the redistribution of DC *in vivo*, as well exemplified by systems of migratory evasion of the T lymphocytes. In specific terms, the ingress of DC cells within tumors is beset by systems for further migratory systems as exemplified by the tumor-draining lymph node lymphocytes.

Resident memory T cells, derived from memory CD8+ T cells, are enriched in tumor specific T cells in close contact with tumor cells and determine the efficacy to cancer vaccines [4].

System Profiles

System profiles of the stressor-related neurohormonal responses recapitulate the directional and polarizing dimensions of response aimed usually towards the tumor antigenicity networks.

Immunosenescence in aging, on the other hand, involves interactivity between immune cell depletion and up-regulation of cytokines [5].

In such terms, the descriptive dimensions of the immune response are foreshadowed by the incremental parameters of the immune response to tumor cells. Deviant pressure -immune exertion is a modulating network in its own right, within system patterns for antigen-processing and presentation by the DC. Foxp3+ regulatory cells determine a balance between immunity and tolerance and their number is negatively regulated by the kinase Lkb1 in DC [6]. Contact dynamics with T lymphocytes expose DC within the system modulations for further antigen-processing and antigen-presentation by DC. The chemokine CCL22 is mainly produced by DC, and it controls T cell immunity by recruiting Tregs to the tumor and by promoting DC-Treg contacts in the lymph nodes [7].

This is an incumbent phenomenon that implicates the derivative nature of the proximal components of the antitumor immune response, as dictated by *in vivo* dynamics of DC that interact with the specific tumor-related milieu of the tumor microenvironment.

RESPONSE MODELS

Models of response inherently incorporate the process of tumor immune escape as projected by incremental dimensions of insufficient potency of the DC processes of maturation. In such terms, the increments in immune response fail to biophysically contact accurately the tumor neoantigens.

The impact of contact dynamics with T lymphocytes is incremental process presentation of antigen within draining lymph nodes. It is further to such consideration that the tumor neoantigenicity fails to be antigen-presented in the lymph nodes and to the specific T lymphocytes.

Current individualised immunotherapy strategies focus on the combined approach that utilises dendritic cell vaccine, adoptive cell therapies such as chimeric antigen receptor T cells and the use of checkpoint inhibitors [8].

INDUCTION

Induction of T lymphocyte response is hence a paramount consideration that is set within the stressor component factors of the tumor microenvironment. In such terms, immune escape of tumor cells is essential conditioning of the immune response, as dictated primarily by DC. The nature of the induction series of phenomena is analogous to the dimensions of migratory functionalities of the DC within a further encompassed milieu of antigen-processing and presentation by the DC. In the overall context of dynamics of the modeled dimensions, tumor cells evade the immune responsiveness as an integral dysfunction that dynamically further modulates DC reactivities.

The significance of such considerations equates the migratory patterns of DC with the malignant tumor spread to draining lymph nodes and to peripheral organs. Tumor necrosis factor-alpha is critical for primary B cell follicles, follicular dendritic cell networks and germinal centers and in the maturation of humoral immune responses [9]. The further postulates of such a process of DC migration determine, in a potent manner, the dimensional scope of malignant tumor cells to spread and form metastatic deposits.

Spread Mechanics

Paramount mechanics of spread of tumor cells are modeled systems of the migratory behavioral patterns as evidenced by DC patterns of reactivity within the T-lymphocyte domains of the draining lymph nodes. It is an incumbent phenomenon that involves the global migration of DC within the profile modeling spread of modulated tumor cells.

Circulating tumor cell fragments generate immune-interacting intermediates and these outline a competitive relationship between various phagocyte populations for tumor loading during metastasis of tumor cells [10]. Incremental biology of DC reactivity is inherent hierarchical dimension as projected by the onset and termination of the antitumor immune response. Dysfunctional appraisal on the part of the integral immune response incorporates tumor escape phenomena, as indeed evidenced often by failed maturation of the DC.

Conclusion

The significance of the immune response to tumor cells is based on a constitutive dysfunctionality of DC within profile mechanistic dimensions of the antigen-presentation by DC. This is proposed within hierarchical systems of modulation of the generic induction phenomenon of the T lymphocytes within the tumor draining lymph nodes.

It is significant to consider processes of degradation of intracellular protein-antigen as DC patterns of initial maturation and homing to the tumor microenvironment. In such terms, ongoing dynamics of spread of tumor cells determine, in specific fashion, the suppression of T lymphocytes, in a manner that substantially incorporates the migratory behavior of the reactive and antigen-loaded DC. Reappraisal mechanics include the contact dynamics of migratory DC with the T-lymphocytic milieu of draining lymph nodes.

REFERENCES

[1] Mami-Chouaib F, Blanc C, Corgnac S, Hans S, Malefic I, Granier C et al. "Resident memory T cells, critical components in tumor immunology" *J Immunother Cancer* 2018;6(1):87.

[2] Padoan A, Plebani M, Basso D "Inflammation and pancreatic cancer: focus on metabolism, cytokines, and immunity" *Int J Mol Sci* 2019;20(3): 676.

[3] Kowal J, Tkach M "Dendritic cell extracellular vesicles" *Int Rev Cell Mol Biol* 2019;349:213-249.

[4] Blanc C, Hans S, Tran T, Garnier C, Saldman A, Anson M et al. "Targeting resident memory T cells for cancer immunotherapy" *Front Immunol* 2018;9:1722.

[5] Ventura MT, Casciaro M, Gangemi S, Buquicchio R "Immunosenescence in aging: between immune cell depletion and cytokine up-regulation" *Clin Mol Allergy* 2017;15:21.

[6] Chen S, Fang L, Guo W, Zhou Y, Yu G, Li W et al. "Control of T(reg) cell homeostasis and immune equilibrium by Lkb1 in dendritic cells" *Nat Commun* 2018;9(1):5298.

[7] Rohrle N, Knott MML, Anz D "CCL22 signaling in the tumor environment" *Adv Exp Med Biol* 2020;1231:79-96.

[8] Van Gool SW, Makalowski J, Fiore S, Sprenger T, Prix L, Schirrmacher V et al. "Randomized controlled immunotherapy clinical trials for GBM challenged" *Cancers* (Basel) 2020;13(1):32.

[9] Pasparakis M, Alexopoulou L, Episkopou V, Kollias G "Immune and inflammatory responses in TNF alpha-deficient mice: a critical requirement for TNF alpha in the formation of primary B cell follicles, follicular dendritic cell networks and germinal centres, and in the maturation of the humeral immune response" *J Exp Med* 1996;184(4):1397-411.

[10] Hadley MB, Bins A, Nip A, Roberts EW, Looney MR, Gerard A et al. "Visualization of immediate immune responses to pioneer metastatic cells in the lung" *Nature* 2016;531(7505):513-7.

Chapter 22

MICROENVIRONMENTAL REPRODUCIBLE IMMUNOMODULATION AS PROPOSED GROWTH AND SPREAD OF MALIGNANT CELLS IN TERMS OF NEOANTIGENICITY

ABSTRACT

System-profile presentation of tumor cell antigenicity is tenet assumption within spheres for further growth and spread of malignant neoplasia. In such terms, the incumbent participation of tumor cell injury is a pro-inflammatory stimulus that arises within the tumor microenvironment in terms of contextual modulation of the possible antitumor immune response. The participation of tumor biologic contexts allows for the emergence and also creation of neoantigenicity as borne out by the profiling modules for further growth of the integral tumor lesion and of spread of the malignant cells. The context for tumor evolutionary change is system redefinition as proposed by participants of the immunomodulatory dimensions that project systemically in terms of the creation and repeated modulation of the tumor microenvironment.

In such terms, the creation of tumor neoantigenicity is system redefinition of range profiles for the integral tumor lesion.

Introduction

The combination of low-dose chemotherapy with immunotherapy in patients with cancer bespeaks for the development of immunomodulatory effects derived from perceived dimensions of immunostimulatory activity against the tumor. In such terms, the ongoing proliferation of tumor cells within the range of low levels of chemotherapy-induced toxicity to normal cells is inhibited in terms that include dendritic cell (DC) immunomodulation. P2X7, a transmembrane receptor, leads to the creation of a macropore and can either drive cell survival and proliferation or induce cell death; its ligand ATP is present in critical amounts in the tumor microenvironment. The incumbent development of stimulatory immune functionality is projected within the tumor microenvironment in a manner that evolves during combinatorial therapy of the low dose chemotherapy and the intralesional injection of DC.

In such terms, the evolving dimensions of stress induced by surgical resection are minimized via mechanisms such as laparoscopic resection of the primary tumor lesion.

Immune checkpoint ligand 1 expressed mainly by T cells, and its ligand (PD-L1) in tumor cells, dendritic cells and macrophages, impede immune function [2].

DC initiates potent antitumor immune responses but may also mediate genomic injury, support neovasculariation and block antitumor immunity [3].

Enhanced Antigen Release

The incumbent approach to the enhanced release of antigens related to tumor cells are stimulatory in terms of a specific series of immunomodulatory systems. MEK inhibition promotes oncolytic virus immunotherapy through increased tumor cell killing and T cell activation

[4]. The development of further stimulation of the immune system is integral to the development of immunotherapeutic approach within the range of significant involvement of tumor neoantigenicity as borne out by dimensions of co-stimulatory molecules and the priming of antigen-specific T lymphocytes.

Immunogenicity of viruses may be harnessed if virus-specific T cells are modified by tumor-specific chimeric antigen receptors [5]. Ongoing production of pro-inflammatory cytokines such as IL-12, and the reduced production of anti-inflammatory cytokines such as IL-10, are inducible indices related to the exposure of tumor cells to very low but sustained levels of chemotherapeutic drugs.

DIMENSIONS OF IMMUNOMODULATION

The release of the dimensionally active immunomodulatory agents is substantial reference to the induction of antigen release by tumor cells in a manner that exacerbates the onset dynamics of primed T-lymphocytes within spheres of ongoing modulation of the antitumor immune response.

Timor-Associated stroll myofibroblasts play a fundamental role in the emergence of an immunosuppressive microenvironment in early prostatic cancer [6].

In such terms, the ongoing evolution of injury to tumor cells is included fractional index of the progressive release of neoantigens within spheres of ongoing mounting of the antitumor immune response.

It is within such referential terms that immunomodulation substantiates the ongoing tumor regression pathways, particularly within the context of such agents as vascular endothelial growth factor (VEGF). VEGF is a central actor within the angiogenesis and immune-suppression encompass as delivered within models of immunomodulation. Autologous T cells directed to the Epstein-Barr virus latent membrane protein 1 and 2 can induce durable complete responses in patients with lymphoma [7].

Recombination Strategies

Substantial recombination strategies that arise within models of immunostimulation are permissive for the emergence of antigenicity that appears unique to malignant tumors, as these infiltrate the microenvironment and spread systematically. In terms of overt dimensions, the emergence of neoantigenicity appear unique to the process of tumor-cell proliferation and spread.

In such terms, the evolutionary course as dimensionalized within spheres of immunostimulation may be considerably enhanced as borne out the system profiles of production of cytokines and chemokines.

Tumor Microenvironment

The tumor microenvironment is symptomatic of a whole series of induced modulatory steps within the trafficking dynamics of incumbent tumor cell biology, as dimensionalized by proliferation of tumor cells that are specifically related to spread of the malignant tumor cells. P2X7 receptor has a central role in the the tutor microenvironment composition due to combined action on ectonucleotidase, ATP release and the immune cell infiltrate [8]. In such terms, ongoing involvement of the tumor-cell neoantigenicity is enhanced participant within the profile models of such cytokines and chemokines. P2X7 plays a pro-inflammatory role in promoting inflammasome formation and release of mature interleukin-1beta by innate immune cells [9].

The incumbent proliferation of tumor cells is thus integral to the evolving participation of tumor-cell biologic emergence of such antigenicity as provoked by the immunomodulatory approach of low but sustained chemotherapeutic agents.

IMMUNOMODULATION

Biologic models of immunomodulation are substantial profile projection as viewed by dimensions of possible further enhancement of the antitumor immune response. In such terms, the evolving tumor biology is variant participant within spheres of the uncontrolled involvement of proliferation and spread of malignant cells.

The evolving context of tumor biologic parameters allows a permissive microenvironment as system profile indices for further growth of the tumor cells and of the integral tumor lesion itself. Activation of P2X7 receptor by ATP enhances breast cancer cell invasion and migration, possibly by the activation of AKT pathway and modulation of E-cadherin and MMP-13 expression [10].

In such terms, ongoing participation of injury to tumor cells is integral to the stimulation of a modulatory immune response that involves substantial modification of neoantigenicity. The injury to tumors and to individual tumor cells is participant profile creation of the immunomodulatory indices of profile projection of systems of emergence of antigen within contextual provocation of the increased tumor cell evolution.

SYSTEM PROFILES

System-profile determination is a cardinal principle as provoked by the emergence of tumor cell neoantigenicity as further proposed by pathways of incumbent production of pro-inflammatory cytokines and chemokines. PWX7 plays a central role in inducing diverse cell responses which upon dysregulation are related to tumor initiation and development [11]. Stimulation of P2X7-Receptor by high levels of ATP leads to cell proliferation, inflammasome activation and the release of extracellular vesicles [12]. P2X7 single-nucleotide polymorphisms may constitute diagnostic biomarkers for tailored therapy [13].

In such context the absorption for evolutionary changes of tumor antigenicity, within shifting polarization of the antigenicity, allows for the production of an immune response that is multi-phasic, as proposed by the operability of the antitumor immunity generated by specific parameters of tumor-cell proliferation and spread.

Conclusion

Profile antigenicity, as proposed by tumor cell proliferation and spread, is distinct from a generic process of antigen exposure in terms of the ongoing immunodulatory activities of the DC profiles of turnover. In terms reminiscent of the viral infections in general, the incumbent evolution of tumor cell dimensions of neoantigenicity is substantial distinction within specifics of a tumor lesion as projected integrally, and as complexed tumor lesions in contextual reference of the host as a whole.

It is significant to view the development of immunomodulatory systems of response as integral networks of a cytokine and chemokine model for further involvement of the host biologic tolerance to the tumor dynamics of cell proliferation and spread.

In such terms, ongoing release of neoantigens is integral participant within the essential modulatory phenomena of the DC system promotion as essential permissive systems for further growth of the integral tumor lesion.

References

[1] Lara R, Adinolfi E, Harwood CA, Philpott M, Barden JA, Di Virgilio F et al. "P2X7 in cancer: from molecular mechanisms to therapeutics" *Front Pharmacol* 2020;11:793.

[2] Macek Jilkova Z, Aspord, Decaens T "Predictive factors for response to PD-1/PD-L1 checkpoint inhibition in the field of hepatocellular carcinoma: current status and challenges" *Cancers* (Basel) 2019;11(10):1554.

[3] Ma Y, Shurin GV, Gutkin DW, Shurin MR "Tumor associated regulatory dendritic cells" *Semin Cancer Biol* 2012;22(4):298-306.

[4] Bommareddy PK, Aspromonte S, Zloza A, Rabkin SD, Kaufman HL "MEK inhibition enhances oncolytic virus immunotherapy through increased tumor cell killing and T cell activation" *Sci Transl Med* 2018;10(471) eau 0417.

[5] Tanaka M, Tashiro H, Omer B, Lapteva N, Ando J, Ngo M et al. "Vaccination targeting native receptors to enhance the function and proliferation of chimeric antigen receptor (CAR)-modified T cells" *Clin Cancer Res* 2017;23(14):3499-3509.

[6] Spary LK, Salimu J, Webber JP, Clayton A, Mason MD, Tabi Z "Tumor stroma-derived factors skew monocyte to dendritic cell differentiation toward a suppressive CD14(+) PD-L1(+) phenotype in prostate cancer" *Oncoimmunology* 2014;3(9):e95533.

[7] Bollard CM, Gottschalk S, Tornado V, Diouf O, Hazrat Y, Carrum G et al. "Sustained complete responses in patients with lymphoma receiving autologous cytotoxic T lymphocytes targeting Epstein-Barr virus latent membrane proteins" *J Clin Oncol* 2014;32(8):798-808.

[8] De Marchi E, Orioli E, Pegoraro A, Sangaletti S, Portararo P, Curti A et al. "The P2X7 receptor modulates immune cells infiltration, ectonucleotidases expression and extracellular ATP levels in the tutor microenvironment" *Oncogene* 2019;38(19):3636-3650.

[9] Rissiek B, Haag F, Boyer O, Koch-Nolte F, Adriouch S "P2X7 on mouse T cells: one channel, many functions" *Front Immunol* 2015;6:204.

[10] Xia J, Yu X, Tang L, Li G, He T "P2X7 receptor stimulates breast cancer cell invasion and migration via the AKT pathway" *Oncol Rep* 2015;34(1):103-10.

[11] Gilbert SM, Oliphant CJ, Hassan S, Peille AL, Bronsert P, Falzoni S et al. "ATP in the tumor microenvironment drives expression of nfP2X7, a key mediator of cancer cell survival" *Oncogene* 2019;38(2):194-208.

[12] Lombardi M, Gabrielli M, Adinolfi E, Verderio C "Role of ATP in extracellular vesicle biogenesis and dynamics" *Front Pharmacy* 2021;12:654023

[13] De Marchi E, Orioli E, Dal Ben D, Adinolfi E "P2X7 receptor as a therapeutic target" *Adv Protein Chem Struct Biol* 2016;104:39-79.

Chapter 23

TUMOR CELL NECROSIS MODULATES THE IMMUNE TOLERANCE INDUCED BY THE TUMOR MICROENVIRONMENT

ABSTRACT

Tumor cell necrosis is recognized participant of the immune responsiveness to the clonogenic expansion of the cancer cells in terms of ongoing signature reformulations of the tumor microenvironment and of its component systems. The mechanisms of participation of system progression as positive feedback formulas allows for the emergence of tolerance immunity as dictated by the performance injury to tumor cells that remodulate the promotional dynamics of the tumor cell necrosis itself. In such terms, ongoing reshaping of the tumor microenvironment constitutes the immuno-suppressive series of responses and nonresponses as growth factors and chemokines respond to immune cell tolerance. It is within such formulas that redefinition of systems of response to tumor cell necrosis acquire permissive attributes of immune suppression and immune tolerance.

Introduction

Dendritic cells (DC) constitute reformulations in terms of the response of the immune system to tumorigenesis, rather than to the established tumor lesion per se. Optimal response to tumor therapy require an intact commensal microbiota that modulates myeloid-derived cell functions within the tumor microenvironment [1]. TNF-alpha, IL-5, TGF-beta, and IL-10, participate in the initiation and progression of cancer, such as generation of reactive oxygen and nitrogen species, mutagenesis and in epithelial mesenchymal transition, angiogenesis and metastasis [2]. In such terms, the ongoing formulas of response of the entire reticulo-endothelial system comprises especially fully functional macrophage subsets. The modulatory roles of systems of antigen recognition are integral to a possible tumor-supporting series of roles of DC and macrophages in the progression of cancer lesions within system profile pathways of ongoing processing and presentation of antigen to T lymphocytes.

The participation of injury to signature formulation of the tumor microenvironment is inherent attribute of the reticulo-endothelial system as presented in terms of immunogenesis. In terms beyond such considerations, antigen presentation is provided pathway series of events that promote distributional systems of chemokine-provoked mobility of the DC, as indeed provided by the reticulo-endothelial system as a whole.

Dendritic Cell Expansion

The incremental dimensions, as expanded DC subsets, is provocative mechanism within the ongoing proposed globality of a cell type that encompasses the transfer of immune components to the reactive immune system.

Necrosis may lead to renewed cancer progression and treatment resistance in the absence of inflammation and involves damage-associated molecular patterns and a pro-cancerous environment [3].

Encompassed redistribution of effects, as DC participation in the creation of immune responsiveness, includes derivative pathways as co-stimulatory molecules, on the one hand, and of a reshaping of the tumor microenvironment. In addition to high levels of intratumoral heterogeneity, glioblastomas also show inter-tumor heterogeneity; correlative data suggest that molecularly distinct glioblastoma subtypes exhibit different microenvironments with their associated macrophages [4]. In such terms, the proportional redistribution of immature DC, within the tumor bed and the predominant localization of mature DC within the tumor microenvironment, allow for the performance of a series of modulatory actions that promote and further propagate immune responsiveness, on the one hand, and of a actuation of proportional support for tumor progression and expansion under certain strict modulating conditions.

Actuation

In a real and actuation series of maneuvers, the substantial reactivity of DC is transferred biology of the mobility mechanisms of the DC, within the further proponent reactivity participation of cell injury and of tumor cell necrosis. Programmed cell death, including apoptosis, autophagy, and necroptosis, are central players in metastatic processes [5]. In such terms, the incremental dimensions of tumor expansion incorporate the realization of pathways established as promoted, and further enhanced, by such systems as bone remodeling and osteoclastic activity. The incumbent participation of tumor cell necrosis is evidential incorporation of tumor cell injury and necrosis, within the scope participation of the reticulo-endothelial system that not only participates in phagocytosis but, above all, is a mobility-enhanced series of signature reformations of the tumor microenvironment. Angiogenic inflammation and necrosis in the tumor microenvironment modulate patient survival after radical surgery [6].

In such terms, ongoing involvement of DC is inherent promotor of both tumor cell recognition, and also, of induced effector immune responsiveness. Whole-genome sequencing, epigenomics and transcriptional profiling have improved prognosis and therapeutic outcome of glioblastoma patients [7].

The corporeality of injury to tumor cells is an essential recovery series of attempts of the injury-responsive pathways that participate with the terms of the incremental immune responsiveness, on the one hand, and of the promoted enhancement of tumor cell injury and its immune recognition. Although tumor-associated macrophages are genetically stable, these can alter their expression profiles in the face of signals from tumor cells; therefore, heterogeneous glioblastomas create heterogeneity in tumor associated macrophages [8]. It is in terms beyond simple participation of immune responsiveness that DC involve, in a substantially significant manner, the participation for further remodeling of the tumor microenvironment.

Immunotherapeutic strategies are aimed to overcome the hurdles of the blood-brain barrier and immunosuppressive tumor microenvironment in glioblastoma patients [9]. The development of injury signature within such tumor microenvironment incorporates the realization of systems of response in adaptive recovery of the tissue injury, that accompanies tumor cell necrosis. In such terms, the ongoing recovery attempts for promotional redistribution of DC subsets incorporate the mobility potentials as proposed by an integral reticulo-endothelial system.

Signature Formulas

Signature formulas, as contributors to the tumor cell necrosis pathways, incorporate the evidential participation of the immune responsiveness that partakes, in actual realistic terms, the significant progression of the tumor lesions. It has been reported that harnessing the cross-talk between glioblastoma cells and tumor-associated macrophages with a nano-drug modulates the glioblastoma immune microenvironment [10].

The participation of such systems of immune recognition reshape a tumor microenvironment in terms of its components as proposed by various growth factors, immune cells and chemokines. Tumor-associated macrophages and microglia are major tumor-promoting immune cells in the tumor microenvironment [11]. The actual integration of such series of cell-injury responses include the reshaping of the immune responses themselves as promulgated by the reshaping modulation of the tumor microenvironment. Single-cell transcriptomics show both tumor and hematopoietic-derived cells in glioblastoma exposed to diverse mediators of immune evasion [12]. In such measure, ongoing redistribution of signature reformulation allow for the re-characterization of the immunity towards the re-performance actions of such components as VEGF-induced angiogenesis, and the conversion of the immune response to a tumor-supporting mechanism of participation.

PERFORMANCE DYNAMICS

Performance dynamics, as a whole system microcosmos series of systems of response, promote the integral further recognition of tumor cell necrosis. 24 immune-related genes have been identified in the tumor microenvironment and 6 of these genes are significantly related to prognosis in glioblastoma patients [13]. The signature reformulations are distribution systems of immune recognition that primarily incorporate the mobility phenomena, as shown by the DC responsive elements. Improved prognostication of glioblastoma has been achieved beyond molecular sub-typing by transcriptional profiling of the tumor microenvironment [14]. In such terms, the incremental progression of tumor cell necrosis is responsible for the expansion of an immune responsiveness within systems of tumor lesion expansion and metastatic spread of the cancer cells.

It is, therefore, in terms of conditional participation of tumor cell necrosis that the tumor microenvironment promotes and further participates as modulation of the tumor cell injury, to enhance the DC support of tumor lesion expansion. Glioblastoma combines a lack of immunogenicity with few mutations and a highly immunosuppressive tumor microenvironment; both tumor and immune cells contribute to this immunosuppression [15].

Conclusion

The performance of tumor injury, as signature enforcement in modulating the immune response, is an incremental system of a positive feedback series of systems within the global and integral reticulo-endothelial system that responses as immune responsiveness to tumor cell necrosis. In such terms, the further enhancement of modulators transform, in simple measure, the redistribution of components of the tumor microenvironment that further conforms to tumor expansion.

The formulas for the performance delivery of growth factors and of tolerance immune components incorporate also chemokine generation as formulated by the modulated immune response. In such measure, the descriptive formulas of the tolerant immune and regulatory cells allow for the permissive emergence as dictated by the re-modeled tumor microenvironment. Systems of re-characterization of the immune response is set integer within the clonogenic proliferation of tumor cells in response to the tumor cell necrosis that promulgates as substance reformation of the signature immune responsiveness of the tumor microenvironment.

REFERENCES

[1] Iida N, Dzutsev A, Stewart CA, Smith L, Bouladoux N, Weingarten RA et al. "Commensal bacteria control cancer response to therapy by modulating the tumor microenvironment" *Science* 2013;342(6161):967-70.

[2] Landskron G, De la Fuente M, Thuwajit P, Thuwajit C, Hermoso MA "Chronic inflammation and cytokines in the tumor microenvironment" *J Immunol Res* 2014;2014:149185.

[3] Karsch-Bluman A, Benny O "Necrosis in the tumor microenvironment and its role in cancer recurrence" *Adv Exp Med Biol* 2020;1225:89-98.

[4] Chen Z, Hambardzumyan D "Immune microenvironment in glioblastoma subtypes" *Front Immunol* 2018;9:1004.

[5] Su Z, Yang Z, Xu Y, Chen Y, Yu Q "Apoptosis, autophagy, necroptosis, and cancer metastasis" *Mol Cancer* 2015;14:48.

[6] Atanasov G, Dino K, Schierle K, Dietel C, Aust G, Pritsche J et al. "Angiogenic inflammation and formation of encores in the tumor microenvironment influence patient survival after radical surgery for de novo hepatocellular carcinoma in non-cirrhosis" *World J Surg Oncol* 2019;17(1):217.

[7] DeCordova S, Shastri A, Tsolaki AG, Yasmin H, Klein L, Singh SK et al. "Molecular heterogeneity and immunosuppressive microenvironment in glioblastoma" *Front Immunol* 2020;11:1402.

[8] Buonfiglioli A, Hambardzumyan D "Macrophages and microglia: the cerberus of glioblastoma" *Acta Neuropathol Cummun* 2021;9(1):54.

[9] Descend FA, Hormigo A "The CNS and the brain tumour microenvironment: implications for glioblastoma immunotherapy" *Int J Mol Sci* 2020;21(19):7358.

[10] Li TF, Li K, Wang C, Liu X, Wen Y, Xu YH et al. "Harnessing the cross-talk between tumor cells and tumor-associated macrophages with a nano-drug for modulation of glioblastoma immune microenvironment" *J Control Release* 2017;268:128-146.

[11] Hutter G, Theruvath J, Graef CM, Zhang M, Schoen MK, Manz EM et al. "Microglia are effector cells of CD47-SIRPalpha antiphagocytic axis disruption against glioblastoma" *Proc Natl Acad Sci USA* 2019;116(3):997-1006.

[12] Close HJ, Stead LF, Nsengimana J, Reilly KA, Droop A, Wurdak H et al. "Expression profiling of single cells and patient cohorts identifies multiple immunosuppressive pathways and an altered NK cell phenotype in glioblastoma" *Clin Exp Immunol* 2020;200(1):33-44.

[13] Huang S, Song Z, Zhang T, He X, Huang K, Zhang Q et al. "Identification of immune cell infiltration and immune-related genes in the tumor microenvironment of glioblastomas" *Front Immunol* 2020;11:585034.

[14] Jeanmougin M, Havik AB, Cekaite L, Brandal P, Sveen A, Meling TR et al. "Improved prognostication of glioblastoma beyond molecular sub-typing by transcriptional profiling of the tumor microenvironment" *Mol Oncol* 2020;14(5):1016-1027.

[15] Pearson JRD, Cuzzubbo S, McArthur S. Durrant LG, Adhikaree J, Tinsley CJ et al. "Immune escape in glioblastoma mutliforme and the adaptation of immunotherapies for treatment" *Front Immunol* 2020;11:582106.

AUTHOR'S CONTACT INFORMATION

Lawrence M. Agius
Department of Pathology (Retired),
Mater Dei Hospital,
University of Malta Medical School,
Msida, Malta
lawrence.agius@um.edu.mt

INDEX

D

E

G

H

I

K

L

S

T

V

W